HEADACHES:

THE DRUGLESS WAY TO LASTING RELIEF!

HEADACHES:
THE DRUGLESS WAY
TO LASTING RELIEF!

HARRY C. EHRMANTRAUT, Ph.D.

CELESTIAL ARTS
BERKELEY, CALIFORNIA

Note to the reader: The purpose of this book is to provide information on headache prevention. It should not be used as a substitute for medical treatment. Anyone with a chronic headache condition would be well advised to consult a physician. If, after undertaking the program featured in this book, serious conditions persist or arise, medical advice should be sought promptly.

CELESTIAL ARTS
P.O. Box 7327
Berkeley, California 94707

Previously published under the same title by Autumn Press, Inc.
Previous edition copyright © 1977, 1980 By Harry C. Ehrmantraut.
Previous ISBN 0–914398–41–5.

Celestial Arts First Printing, 1987

Cover design by Ken Scott
Interior design by Paul Reed
Composition by QuadraType, San Francisco
Interior illustrations by Walt Wedlock

Library of Congress Cataloging-in-Publication Data

Ehrmantraut, Harry C., 1921–
    Headaches: the drugless way to lasting relief.

    Bibliography: p. 129
    Includes index.
    1. Headache—Prevention—Popular works. I. Title.
[DNLM: 1. Headache—therapy—popular works.
WL 342 E33h]
RB128.E38   1987   616.07'2   80–66697
ISBN 0-89087-490-5

Manufactured in the United States of America

1 2 3 4 5 — 91 90 89 88 87

Table of Contents

Part II: Curing Your Headache

CONTENTS

Preface

My own headaches began many years ago. Since then I have read most of the books that have been written about headaches, and, while informative, they have almost all followed a pattern that has both puzzled and frustrated me. Generally, 80 to 90 percent of each book is devoted to detailed descriptions of various types of headaches, outlining all of the various symptoms and side effects, with a bare chapter at the end suggesting some drugs for relief, or recommending some of the many headache clinics that have been formed in recent years. But in terms of specific suggestions as to what the headache victim can do, nothing.

My approach is different. It is clear that the pain in all headaches arises from the same problem, and that problem can be prevented, *provided:* that you are willing to work at it!

Subsequent chapters will discuss tension, migraine, and other headaches in some detail for those of you who wish to classify your problems more clearly, but an in-depth understanding of this is not necessary for the prevention of your headaches. It is far more important that you fully understand the way that pain is generated in headaches, and the nature of pain in general, than it is to worry about the detailed definitions of headache types. My objective is to prevent your headaches. My system has kept me free of headaches for years and will do the same for you.

PART I

You and Your Headache

CHAPTER 1

The Head

If we are to understand fully the nature and cause of head-aches, a general knowledge of the structure and organization of the head itself is essential. The head, of course, is an extremely complex part of the body, but we are concerned basically with the muscles and blood vessels, all external to the skull, that are illustrated in this section. The chief artery of interest is the temporal artery, especially the so-called superficial branch.

On both sides of the head this artery ascends from the neck, below and in front of the ears, proceeds upward directly in front of the ears, then angles forward and upward to the upper temple area, from which it divides widely over the forehead.

The temporal artery is the prime culprit in a large percentage of headaches, and many of you will immediately associate the above description of its location with your own description of headache pains. Remember especially the "in front of the ear" and the "upper temple" areas, and you will see the relation to much of the massage and brushing technique.

The second most important artery is the occipital artery, which arises from beneath and behind the ears on each side of the head and divides inward from each side across the lower back of the skull. Again, you will recognize the location relative to many tension headache pains.

The prime muscles of interest also fall into front and rear

groups. In the frontal group, although really at the side of the head, is the temporalis muscle, covering that key area in front of and above the ear. As you can see, it covers a wide area along the side of the skull and attaches to the lower jaw. Place your fingers along a line between the top of your ear and corner of your eyebrow, and now clench your teeth lightly. That is the temporalis muscle that you feel moving under your fingertips. When talking to someone, experts in body language will always look for signs of contraction and/or motion in this muscle, as it often expresses inner tension. One of the key objectives of our program is to keep this temporalis muscle calm and relaxed.

The frontalis muscle covers the front of the head and forehead like a cap, and is the muscle that raises the eyebrows or moves the scalp forward. Again, it is important to remember because it occupies an area of pain. The remaining muscles of interest in the front are those surrounding the eyes, which interact with the frontalis. Since they are very complex, we will not discuss them in detail, but just ask that you be aware of their interaction with the frontalis and temporalis.

The last area is the back of the head, and here we have first the occipitalis, which really is a continuation of the frontalis, just opposite it. It covers the lower back of the skull and, in most of us, does very little moving. It is important, however, because of its location, and because the occipital artery lies embedded in it. Of next importance is a wide group of muscles that connect the rear base of the skull with several of the upper vertebrae of the spinal column, overlying and supporting one another in action as they flex, rotate, and hold the head. One of these smaller muscles also connects to your shoulder blades.

Overlying all of these is the most important muscle in tension headaches, the trapezius. This very large muscle gives much of the shape to our shoulders. Notice on the illustration that its origin is the "external occipital protuberance." To locate these protuberances, place the middle finger of each hand into the center of each ear. Now move that finger directly behind the ear, on each side, at the same level, and feel for the rounded knob that sits about two inches to each side of the midline. Those are the protuberances, and they are very important to your headaches. Not in themselves, because skull bones do not cause headaches, but because of the muscles that are attached to them. The areas from these bones to the tops of your shoulder blades are the truly vital areas for tension headaches, far and away the most common form of headache, and one that is very often a contributing culprit even in migraines.

The trapezius muscle may be thought of as consisting of three portions: upper, middle, and lower sections. You will note that overall it is triangular, with the broad base of the triangle running up and down along the spine. The middle and lower parts of the muscle originate along the vertebrae of the spine and run over the shoulder blade, attaching to it near the shoulder. These parts are often involved in tension in the back and shoulders, but the prime culprit in headaches is the upper section, running directly from the skull to the shoulder blade. Shrug your shoulders, and you can feel this muscle tense and lift the shoulders. Tensing one trapezius, instead of both, will draw the head to one side. Locking the shoulders in position and then tensing both will pull the head back. Many shoulder and neck motions are included in our exercise section, primarily because of the "traps," as body-builders call the trapezius.

We have talked of "body language" before, and again, shoulder position and elevation speak loud and clear. These muscles seem to be particularly attached to our instincts. Is there one among us who, if suddenly caught in a rain shower, will not immediately and automatically hunch his or her shoulders? This reaction persists even if we are wearing rain gear or carrying an umbrella. Also, with almost all of us, if we get "uptight," the parts which go "up" right away are the shoulders. How? By contracting the "traps," and, what's worse, by *keeping* them contracted, pulling on the protuberances, impinging on the pain sensors in the muscle tissue, and pressing on the occipital artery we discussed above. No wonder you work yourself into a headache!

"Headache" Arteries & Muscles

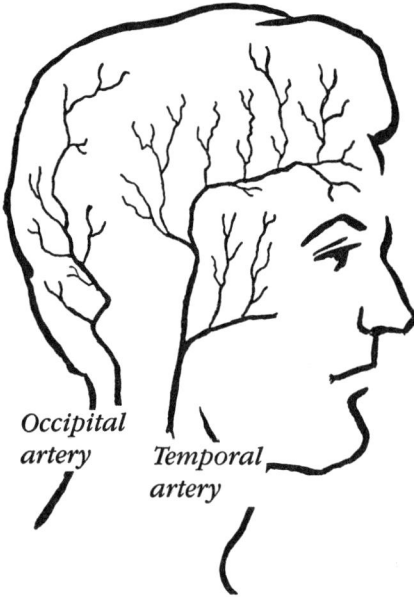

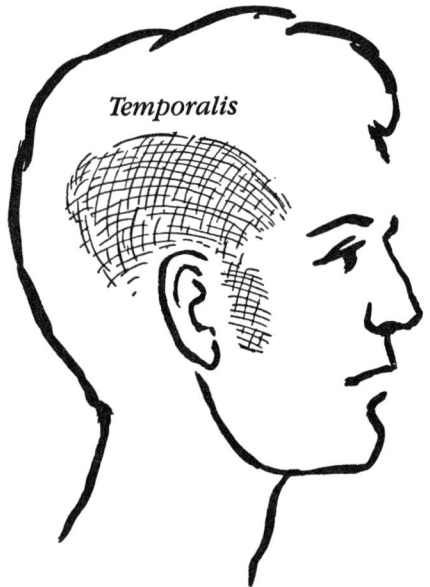

Occipital
artery   Temporal
artery

Temporalis

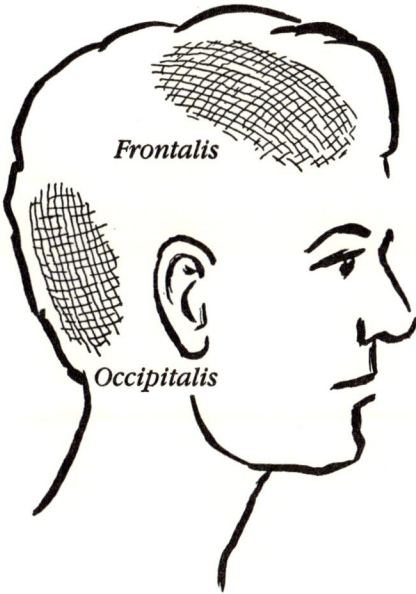

Frontalis

Occipitalis

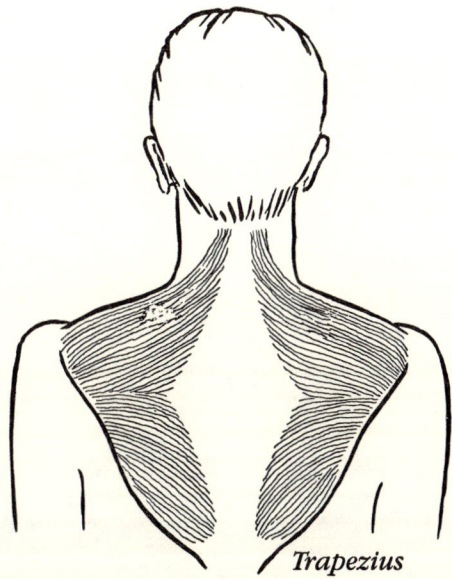

Trapezius

CHAPTER 2

Pain

The Nature of Pain

It is not necessary that you become an expert on all the types and variations of headaches; such knowledge provides little basis for cure and prevention, unless you have a very specific problem such as allergy headaches. However, it is very useful to have a real understanding of the nature of pain, its causes, purposes, manifold varied aspects, and, of course, its prevention.

Detailed studies of pain began back in the late 1800s, when both psychology and physiology were strongly involved in sensory perception. The special nerve endings involved in seeing and hearing were matched by the discovery of special nerves on the skin in localized spots, so that some minute areas would respond to cold, some to warmth, some to touch, while some produced pain. Microscopic examination of the skin showed special nerve endings of different shapes that produced the special sense response, except that the pain impulses seemed to arise from plain naked nerve endings. Not so surprising if one stops to think that the simplest form of pain (known scientifically as "irritability") is a basic characteristic of all protoplasm, shown by amoebae and other unicellular life.

One assumption, then, from an evolutionary view, would be

that the specialized nerve ending developed later as animals grew more complex, but the old basic nerve ending hung on throughout evolution, still delivering pain messages. It is a basic characteristic of nerve fibers that they can transmit only one message; that is, they are essentially "on" or "off." If a nerve ending in the retina of the eye is stimulated by something other than light (for example, electrically, or by pressure at the back of the eyeball), the brain will still perceive that stimulus as a flash of light.

Thus the early "specificity theory" of pain, in which pain was understood as only the stimulation of free nerve endings, was developed. However, about the same time, the "pattern theory" of pain was conceived, which suggested that the feeling of pain was due to a summation of a number of nerve fiber inputs, so that some critical level must be reached before any sensation of pain will arise. In this theory, the brain becomes a major factor in summing and sifting the nerve inputs.

The "gate control theory" most satisfactorily explains the current facts known about pain and pain perception. It uses the facts known about two neural conducting systems in the spinal cord: one tells the brain where and how strong the pain input is; the second is concerned with the interpretation of the pain—the suffering. The first (or basic pain information) is carried in small fibers; the second (or suffering information) is carried in large fibers, and these latter fibers can strongly influence the brain's perception of the inputs from the small fibers. If those large fibers are artificially stimulated, say electrically, they can completely block the transmission from the small fibers, thus preventing the reception of the pain impulse.

In addition to the nerve aspects of pain, you should be aware of the chemical mediators; these are vitally important in headache pain. In many types of pain, it is a chemical that actually stimulates the nerve endings, and *this is certainly the case with your headaches.* One could list chemicals such as bradykinin, histamine, etc., which are all produced by the body and which cause pain sensations, but let's look at a simple illustration you will immediately accept. All of us have suffered at some time the pain coming after strenuous physical exertion. Depending on the sport, exercise, or work you may have felt very specific pain from some muscle area—a bicep, a forearm, perhaps a calf or thigh muscle. This is a classic example of pain from a chemical your body has produced itself.

Nothing strange or foreign is involved here, only your own body biochemistry. Headaches are no different.

This concept is basic to your headaches. To help you understand it fully, let me describe a commonly used technique of producing pain in subjects in the laboratories where pain is studied. It is called "ischemic" pain (ischemia being the medical term for lack of blood in a given part of the body) because of the way it is induced. The subject raises one arm, to drain most of the blood, and the arm is wrapped with an elastic bandage from the hand down to the elbow to further drain the blood vessels. Then a blood pressure cuff is placed just above the elbow and inflated so no further arterial blood can enter the forearm. At this point there is no pain, because simply removing blood from the tissue does not create pain. Now the subject's arm is unwrapped (there still is no pain), and he is asked to squeeze a loaded resistance device with that hand, to have the muscles perform work (and in the process of doing work produce waste metabolic products). A modest amount of work is enough. Now, after a quiet wait, pain will develop as the waste products begin to reach the nerve endings, slowly at first but steadily building to an unbearable level.

Release of the cuff to permit the flow of blood and the flushing out of the waste products will instantly reduce and then eliminate the pain. Do you see an immediate relationship to your headaches?

We will discuss this in more detail later. These chemical pains can be mediated by many means, including aspirin, which acts directly on the chemical-sensing sites; morphine and narcotics, which act on the higher centers where the pain impulses are perceived; and various methods that are effective through the gating control systems described above.

My system uses several approaches to prevent such pain. First, it reduces muscle tension and increases circulation so that very little buildup of these metabolic waste products can occur. Second, it reduces your perception of the pain impulses even if the pain endings are activated. For example, it has recently been shown (in work at UCLA) that acupuncture produces part of its pain-relieving effects by stimulating the release of natural chemical painkillers that are produced normally in each person's body. These natural substances, and narcotics such as morphine, act on the same centers in the brain. Thus, the acupressure methods detailed later in this book reduce your headache pain just as effectively as the strongest of painkillers, but without the hazards and side effects.

Paradox of Pain

There are several paradoxes associated with pain, the most basic being its conflicting beneficial and harmful qualities. There are individuals born with an abnormality that leaves them with no sense of pain whatsoever. Medical history shows that they are doomed to an endless chain of injuries from burns and other sources, aggravation of sprains or breaks, and in several cases death from appendicitis, because no warning abdominal pain was felt.

Pain can indeed be harmful, especially long-term unremitting pain, which can shatter an individual's morale to the point of literally not caring whether he lives or dies. A headache victim may live in such dread of the next attack that even during periods of well-being he feels pursued by some unseen assailant who may strike at the most unexpected, and often most inopportune, time.

Moreover, pain is a complex entity. Attorneys are apt to describe their plaintiff's loss as due to the trilogy of "pain, suffering, and mental anguish." In a very real sense, pain and suffering are two related, but by no means identical, quantities. In the simple example of chemically induced pain, such as the pain of sore muscles, this may in fact not only produce no suffering, but indeed produce a marvelous sense of accomplishment and well-being, even though we are still very aware of the pain arising from the tired muscles.

An extreme example of the separation of pain and suffering would be the medical histories of prefrontal lobotomies performed for the relief of intractable pain. The patients frequently stated that the same pain was there as before the operation, but that they were no longer bothered by it. Morphine and related drugs appear to act primarily by reducing suffering rather than pain, as do the various tranquilizers.

Another way to highlight the difference between pain and suffering is to consider the kinds of situations with which we are all familiar that produce suffering without pain. For example, being in a room that is too warm or too cool can produce great discomfort with absolutely no pain, as can a very "stuffy" room or certain unpleasant odors. Obviously some odors, such as tear gas, can produce both pain and discomfort, but others, such as strong garlic, which may be mouth-watering to some, may cause total discomfort to others, even though no trace of pain exists. If this all sounds academic, please consider that in the case of your own headache problems, you truly would not care about a little residual pain if you could totally eliminate your suffering.

We talked above about the informational aspect of pain, the small nerve fibers that told us just where the pain was. However, there are broad classes of pain where the nerve inputs give us no information, or very misleading information, as to where the pain is located. Three main classes are "phantom limb" pain, "referred" pain, and "psychosomatic" pain.

Phantom limb pain arises where there has been an amputation, but quite commonly the patient will feel that the foot or limb is still there, and can feel pains apparently originating from that part of the body. Nor is the pain terminated by numbing the stump end with local anesthetics in some cases. Evidently the pain is carried in some sort of memory bank, to be recalled later but perceived as present pain. This may have great relevance to the headache victim who has sudden headaches at "inconvenient" (but perhaps socially convenient) times.

Referred pain is that pain felt by the patient to be in one part of the body, often a very specific spot, but actually arising from a different part. An example would be the shooting pains of the upper leg that actually originate in the sacroiliac region of the lower back, or the upper arm and shoulder pains associated with most heart attacks.

Psychosomatic pains are those arising without organic basis in the body, but caused by emotional stresses and the individual's reaction to those stresses; but let there be no confusion or doubt in your mind that these are *real* pains, as real to the victim as any other kind, and just as deserving of treatment.

The above paragraphs emphasize the paradox of pain, not only the plus and minus of feeling pain, but that the information the victim's own brain receives about the location and nature of his pain must be examined carefully and interpreted with due caution.

Source of Pain

To understand this system of headache prevention, you need to understand the source of your headache pain: where, exactly, does the pain start?

The first thing to understand is that *the pain does not come from your brain.* The brain itself is insensitive and, in fact, even cutting it will not produce pain. Second, it is very unlikely that the pain comes from within the cranium at all. (The cranium consists of those skull bones surrounding the brain.) The only elements inside the cranium that can sense pain are parts of the blood vessels and the parts of the brain-covering membranes immediately adjacent to these blood vessels. Thus, only two problems *within* the cranium can cause headache pain, and neither of these is the cause in even 1 percent of the headaches of the general population.

One of these problems is a brain tumor that is sufficiently advanced in size to actually pull or press on a sensitive part of the membrane or blood vessel. Usually by this time, the tumor will have produced other effects, such as vision problems, dizziness, etc., long before it produces headaches. The second source is sudden and violent accelerations of the head, especially in rotation, so that the mass of the brain, continuing to turn slightly after the skull has stopped, will pull on the main arteries at its base.

In over 99 percent of headaches, the pain comes from outside of your skull. In fact, it originates in the tissues lying outside of the skull and under the skin, namely the muscles and blood vessels of the scalp and neck. The actual source of pain is the end of the pain nerve. That pain nerve terminates in one of three structures: the large and small skeletal muscles of the neck; the small muscles making up the scalp; or the very small muscles comprising the walls of the arteries and veins of the scalp, forehead, and neck. *All of your headache pain comes from nerve endings in muscles.*

This is an extremely fortunate fact for headache victims. If the pain arose from the brain, it would be very difficult to reach, to manipulate, and to control. But as this pain arises totally from muscle tissue which we clearly *can* reach and manipulate, we *can* control it. The pain is sensed because the bare ends of the pain nerves are irritated. Any irritation will give rise to pain, since that is the only message these nerves can convey, but the usual irritation is either *mechanical* or *chemical.*

Mechanical irritation arises from the muscle being contracted tightly for some period of time (this compresses the nerve ending), from exterior pressure on the muscle, or by stretching of the muscle fibers. Thus, the pain endings in the wall of the artery can be irritated if the muscles of the wall relax too much, permitting the pressure of the blood to stretch the wall until the whole artery is distended.

Chemical irritation arises from a wide variety of natural substances produced in the body that are normally kept below irritant level by the flushing action of the circulation system. The metabolic waste products of exercise in a muscle can be very painful if their normal removal is prevented. These and other natural substances circulating can also have a powerful effect on certain chemicals (so-called amines) in the brain, which control the level at which irritation of the nerve endings is perceived by the brain as pain. In other words, your pain threshold is actually adjusted up and down by these circulating chemicals. On those days when you think you are a little more "touchy" to the normal irritations of life, you may actually be more touchy to pain itself.

In general, pain is sensed in the area from which the pain signal is sent. Occasionally, however, it will be sensed in a somewhat different area, or over a much wider area than is actually being irritated. For this reason, my system directs your attention not only to the specific places where you feel your headaches, but to all of the headache areas.

Since the pain comes from muscles, whether large or small, the next question is: why are the muscles causing pain? The answer: because these particular muscles have lost their proper muscle tone. Muscle tone is a term used to describe the normal state of contraction of the muscles when they are not being specifically activated for motion: some muscle fibers alternately contract and relax, maintaining a moderate degree of tension in the muscle. This "tone" is a function not only of the muscle itself, but of the motor nerves running to and controlling the muscle. Too much tone, and the muscle is contracted and under continual stress; too little tone, and the muscle is overrelaxed and flaccid. Like many things in life, and most certainly in the body, the proper balance between too much and too little is the key.

The whole secret of eliminating headaches is to normalize the tone of all the muscles, large and small, of the head and neck.

Control of Pain

It has been shown experimentally that dogs raised in a specially restricted environment of "sensory deprivation" have no sense of pain and are very slow to learn a pain response even when later exposed to painful stimuli. Obviously there is a large "learned" component in what we simply call pain. Tests using uniform pain stimuli have shown that there are large differences in this learned component. Children from larger families complain of pain more readily than children from small families. Is this a necessary reaction to the problem of getting noticed in a large group? Also, ethnic backgrounds show marked differences in apparent response to pain. The typically outspoken Italian and Jewish cultures seem to feel freer to verbalize pain, demonstrating lower tolerances in a given circumstance, while the Nordic and Teutonic groups have more restrained reactions to pain. This does not suggest any differences in the amount of pain persons from a given background can stand, only what their customary reaction to pain might be.

We are all familiar with the image of pain tolerance that books, movies, and now television have created: the tough frontiersman or cowboy, walking or riding across the plains with a broken leg, or the stoic Indian rubbing mud on the wound from the white man's gun and riding back to the charge—or the secret agent refusing to talk even when the laser beam burns the soles of his feet. Ridiculous? Ah, but not so ridiculous, when you wonder why people seem ashamed of pain, when you wonder why some headache victims are embarrassed to be put out of action by something as niggling as a headache. The ability to withstand pain is an old cultural attribute sometimes still carried over into initiation ceremonies.

Nor is this all bad. The ability of a person to drive himself on under conditions of physical discomfort or even real pain not only has strong survival benefits under certain circumstances, but the kind of emotional and mental toughness that ignores pain and suffering may yield the kind of drive necessary to fulfill Edison's famous definition of genius: "5 percent inspiration and 95 percent perspiration." The key word in that last sentence is "may"; indeed it may lead to it, or be transferable, but not necessarily. The premise of the Outward Bound programs is that a young person develops self-confidence in stressful situations in the wilderness that will carry over into everyday life. And well they may. But we are all different individuals, with different strengths and resources. I have seen the self-reliant outdoors type fail miserably in a business situation that he could not attack in the same physical manner, while some city slicker ran off with the prize.

It is also vital to keep in mind that while generally pain might be considered punishment, it can be a very rewarding experience, given the right set of circumstances. The oft-laughed-at "nighttime headache" as a way for the wife to avoid sex is but one of a multitude of examples of pain as an excuse. Think for a moment of our common evaluation of depression versus an injured back. If an employee came to you and said, "I'm really depressed this afternoon; I don't think I can work; I'd better go home," your reaction would be either to order him to go back to work or to look for another job, or at least to put some very large question marks against this employee in your mental file. But if he came in and said, "I'm really in a lot of pain from my back," you almost surely would give him the rest of the day off.

All of us have faced situations in life where an illness, not too serious but serious enough to remove us totally from the problem, would seem very attractive. A very large fraction of headaches fits this very description.

To fully understand "control *of* pain," one must also consider "control *by* pain." Pain and its companion, suffering, have been controlling factors in the lives of most of us at one time or another. Many of us, as children, were controlled at home by the direct application or threat of pain. At school, the threats of pain and suffering were a constant method of control. Certainly there was no pain involved in staying after school or being dressed down in front of the whole class, but there was a whole lot of suffering in some cases. And remember, we continually mix pain and suffering in sensing our personal well-being. Is it any wonder that some headache-prone individuals can create headaches for themselves merely by thinking intensely about some past period when they had great suffering, even if that suffering may have initially been totally pain free? Can you see why job or social or family situations that produce suffering can also produce headaches?

To get to a more detailed discussion of control of pain, let us break it into four categories—physical, drugs, surgery, and psychological—and briefly cover each.

Physical: This would include such approaches as hot and cold treatments, massage, traction, acupuncture and acupressure, electrical stimulation, counterirritants, and audioanalgesia. This book contains detailed sections on several of the physical methods that I feel are particularly applicable, so I will not discuss those here. A few words about audioanalgesia may be constructive because it illustrates several of the interrelations of pain and suffering. Some of you may have experienced this analgesia at your dentist's office, since it has been more popular there, perhaps, than in other applications. Of course, the earphones by themselves reduce the emotional effect of the drill sound slightly, but experiments have shown that a "white noise" background is most effective. White noise has been described as similar to a fragmented wind noise, or a kind of hissing sound. When coupled with music, this is very effective with some patients. However, research has shown clearly that the sound has no analgesic effect on the patient unless the *suggestion* is made to the patient that this will reduce his pain perception and discomfort. Clearly this method is a combination of physical and psychological effects.

Drugs: Probably the earliest was alcohol, since various fermented drinks appear in almost all primitive societies. It probably works more on suffering than on pain itself, and in certain headaches can increase the pain because of its dilating (enlarging) effects on the blood vessels of the scalp.

Aspirin is discussed in a separate section, along with the now common aspirin substitutes. I will only say here that it works directly on the sensor of the pain, and that with most headache victims it also has a large placebo effect; i.e., often the headache will be at least partially relieved before the aspirin could ever have been dissolved and absorbed!

Morphine and other narcotics, both natural and synthetic, act primarily on the brain centers where pain is perceived, reducing the suffering component more than the pain itself. Since morphine and such narcotics should *never* be used for headaches, the only point in discussing them here is as a general review of pain control. But I would like to point out that even with so vigorous a painkiller as morphine, the placebo effect is still very strong. (A placebo is an inert substitute, such as a sugar pill or a saline solution, presented to the patient as a drug.) In studies of the relief of postoperative pain it has been shown that about one-third of the patients will get more relief from morphine than from the placebo; about one-third will get the same relief from the placebo as from the morphine; and about one-third will get very little relief from either the morphine or the placebo.

One last comment about drugs involves the effects of chemical nerve blocks. This involves injecting a local anesthetic in and around a nerve bundle so that the transmission of the nerve impulses is blocked. Even with a local anesthetic that has a numbing effect lasting only minutes, the nerve block may eliminate the pain as perceived by the patient for days or even weeks. Apparently the drug is able to interrupt some kind of vicious circle of self-sustaining pain and thus long outlast its immediate effect on the nerve. This is very relevant to some of the nondrug methods we will discuss later for alleviating the discomfort of a headache.

Surgery: Since the pain is transmitted over nerve fibers, and then processed by certain centers in the brain, the pain can be eliminated by cutting either the fibers bringing the signal in or the center that processes it. This is generally done at one of three kinds of locations, either (1) cutting the roots of sensory nerves outside of the spinal cord, (2) cutting tracts of the spinal cord itself, or (3) cutting parts of the brain itself. Of course, all of these are *drastic* measures, only to be even considered after *all* other approaches have been taken, and only described here because even this drastic approach is *not* always successful. Sometimes the pain is reduced for a time only to build back to the original levels, again confirming the thesis that pain and suffering are very complex phenomena. You must be willing to work at solving your headache problems, the most important factor in this work being *consistency.*

Psychological: These would include behavior modification, relaxation techniques, and biofeedback, the latter two being discussed in other parts of this book. The important aspect of behavior modification, especially the method known as operant conditioning, is that it works by reinforcing the desired action. We are all familiar with training our dog by rewarding certain acts, either with a "doggy yummy" or simply by praise and pats. He then does what earns him praise. In our own case, we may do what earns *us* sympathy. And there is a key danger with headaches: are we somehow rewarded when we have a headache? Sounds silly? Stop and think back to some of your headaches: when they occurred, the circumstances, who was involved, the effect on immediate personal circumstances, etc. There is no doubt now that much illness is emotionally caused, and we will discuss this more in the section on holistic medicine. What makes headaches so attractive as the illness mechanism is that they are safe; no one ever died of a headache. But what a convenient excuse!

I am not claiming that your headaches are phony, or just an excuse imagined to avoid doing something unpleasant. Far from it; your headaches are *very* real, even if they fit some of the psychological descriptions mentioned above. They are *very* painful, and we still intend to cure them. But thinking about the above concept will be helpful in achieving that cure.

CHAPTER 3

The Causes of Headaches

Tension Headaches

This is the most important class of headache to the general public for the simple reason that 90 percent of our headaches are tension headaches. Unless your headaches fit the brief description under migraines, or the other types of headaches, you, too, almost certainly suffer tension headaches. And that is GOOD NEWS for you, since tension headaches can most certainly be totally prevented, if you are willing to work at your problem.

Regardless of where you may sense them at first, these headaches usually start at the rear of the head, eventually radiating forward to involve both sides of the head (although perhaps not with equal intensity). Sometimes they advance to a temple or to just behind the eyes, often so encompassing the head that the victim describes the sensation as having a "tight band around the head" or "like my head was caught in a vise." Unlike migraines, these strike men as frequently as women, perhaps more so.

"Tension headaches" are most aptly named, on both the physical and emotional levels. The immediate source of the pain is tension in the muscles of the neck, shoulders, and skull. In turn, that tension usually, but not always, arises from emotional tension in the victim's personal life situation. The exceptions to this rule would be the purely physical tension brought on by lengthy postural stresses, such as bending over a desk, drafting board, or typewriter, and similar working positions.

As a general rule, it is safe to say that a tension headache is precipitated by tension in the immediate life situation. This may arise from anger, aggravation, frustration, guilt, or related emotional states. Typical is the "fight or flight" reaction, where a stimulus causes the adrenaline to flow, the pulse to race, the body to come alert so that we can either fight the intruder or flee to safety. But in our modern world, we rarely do either. If the "intruder" is our boss, we respond carefully and in a measured way, certainly maintaining our point of view, but perhaps not quite as vigorously as we would like. If the "intruder" is an employee, our husband or wife, our son or daughter, or whatever, there are almost always reasons that we temper our response, ease the intensity of our thrust. The energy was initiated by the intrusion, but if we cannot release it fully, where does it go? All too often, it goes directly into contracting the muscles of the shoulders and neck.

Perhaps at first you will question my description of the tension headache as being a reaction to an immediate life situation. You may well realize that a given headache had its origin in an affront you suffered two weeks ago from your son-in-law, or your mother-in-law, or when you were passed over for promotion three months ago. But stop and review: you haven't had a headache constantly since that intrusion into your life. So the immediacy is incurred in the conscious review of that initial event in your mind. Perhaps you were suddenly reminded of it, and it began to play back through your mind like a bad dream. That replay is the immediate instigator of your headache; as real as far as your gut reaction to it as if it had just occurred.

Tension headaches are often a continuing problem for those individuals who have difficulty expressing their anger. Keeping anger "bottled up" is an apt metaphor for this problem: as the cork is pushed down into the bottle, the head is pulled down into the shoulders. Sex is often another source, ranging from the Victorian type who may be plagued by some type of guilt, to the swinging playboy who puts himself under tremendous pressure to perform, worrying about "making it" in the current culture.

Depression, one of the most common problems of American life, is another prevalent source of tension headaches. In this vicious circle, the depressed person worries endlessly about the very fact of his depression, and the resulting headaches reinforce the feeling of worthlessness inherent in the depression. In milder forms, this is often the source of weekend and holiday headaches, particularly among strongly motivated individuals who may either feel guilty about taking time off from their success-oriented patterns, or, given the time to consider, find their achievements to date lacking. It may be said, with a large element of truth, that *all of us who are headache victims may simply take life too seriously.*

The usual medical approach to tension headaches is the "analgesic and tranquilizer" route; the former to raise the pain threshold, the latter to lower muscle tension. Repeated controlled studies with many patients have shown placebos (pills made of sugar or other inert matter) to have about equal effect when administered with the proper suggestions as to their effectiveness. Clearly, it is the *suggestion* that is effective.

Fortunately, there are also many physical methods that are truly effective for tension headaches, and we will concern ourselves with these very intensively in later sections. Followed consistently, these techniques will totally end tension headaches.

Migraines

Migraine headaches are only the second most common type, following tension headaches, but they are at the top of the list of one who has them. Indeed, many migraine victims are seriously victimized just by the *fear* that they will have an attack.

Do you have migraines? Well, many headaches fit in the gray area between definitions, and also many headaches involve both migraine and tension aspects. The classic definition of a migraine usually involves headaches associated with two of the following: (1) unilateral pain, (2) visual aura, (3) nausea or vomiting, (4) family history of migraine, or (5) previous attacks of vomiting.

Some physicians would weigh heavily the periodicity of the headaches; e.g., the patient who has headaches only on weekends (or, perhaps more specifically, only on Saturdays) would certainly be considered a likely migraineur.

The unilateral pain, of course, refers to the one-sidedness of the pain, often in the forehead and temporal area, and in and around the eye on that side.

The visual aura refers to a wide variety of visual oddities that almost always precede the migraine. These may vary from apparent flashes of light to "holes" or "blanks" in the visual field, to hallucination-type effects, to the odd sensation that anything looked at appears "etched" against its background. Coupled with this is usually a great sensitivity to bright light, especially direct sunlight.

The nausea and vomiting is perhaps not quite as common as the aura, but occurs in a large number of cases, and is a confirming element in the identification of migraine headaches.

The family history aspect is a little suspect to me, for several reasons. Since migraines tend to diminish and disappear in middle age, many patients do not have a clear recollection of their parents' problems during the most relevant age periods. And because of the difficulties of identifying headache types even in the immediate parent, the problems of carrying this identification back a generation or two become enormous.

Classically, the migraineur has been considered very likely to be a specific personality type: intelligent, ambitious, strongly motivated, hard-working, very restrained and well disciplined. Physically, they were thought to be light-boned and lightly muscled, gracefully slim, and active people. The headaches typically start between the ages of fifteen and thirty-five, and occur about twice as often in women as in men. In women, the episodes are often linked with the menstrual period.

The headache often comes on very swiftly after the visual effects, and may last from twelve to even seventy-two hours. During this period, the pain may be only a dull aching sensation, but for most victims it is a severe, often prostrating, pain, which the migraineur comes to absolutely dread. He or she may live in constant fear that the initial symptoms may reappear, knowing only too well the suffering that will follow.

The pattern, however, is not always consistent; pain may switch from one side to the other, or become all-encompassing; time periods or sequence may change from one attack to the next; some patients may feel all the symptoms except the headache at times.

Self-help methods to end the pain range from full body and vigorous exercise for some victims to complete bedrest (usually in a dark room) for most. Caffeine, in the form of strong tea or coffee, has helped many. Of course, a wide range of prescription drugs is available, of which ergotamine is the oldest and most widely used, and new ones appear with regularity. However, they all seem to succeed in a modest percentage of cases, and fail in a goodly percentage. Cold towels and icepacks are often used, and some success has been reported from inverted position, i.e., standing on one's head.

The most important fact from the research and clinical literature on migraines is the establishment that the cause of the pain in migraines is the distention of the extracranial arteries. In other words, the walls of the arteries around the sides of the skull, beneath the skin and scalp, are being stretched by the pressure of the blood flow in them and are creating pain from the walls of those vessels. This problem and its solution are discussed in great detail later in this book, but be certain that you understand that *the pain arises because of incorrect muscle tone in the muscular walls of these blood vessels.*

Hypoglycemia

If you frequently have morning headaches (upon arising or shortly thereafter), or if you have them consistently in the late afternoon, you should consider the possibility that you are hypoglycemic. In an oversimplified sense, hypoglycemia is the opposite of diabetes. However, it has been estimated that one person in every ten is hypoglycemic, so it is certainly worth reviewing here.

In addition to the headaches arising some hours after your last intake of food, typical symptoms may include unusual fatigue and exhaustion, dizziness, drowziness, insomnia in which you awake from a sound sleep but can't go back to sleep, irritability and nervousness, anxiety and/or depression, phobias or thoughts of suicide, tremors and cold sweats, and muscle pains or leg cramps. Obviously not all of these will occur in the usual victim, but any combination of the above with your headaches should be checked out.

Hypoglycemia is a condition in which the body's balancing mechanism for maintaining normal blood sugar levels does not operate properly. Since our brains are very sensitive to the concentration of glucose (simple sugar) in the bloodstream, an abnormally low level will induce many of the above effects. In diabetes, the blood sugar tends to rise sharply above normal levels; in hypoglycemia, the blood sugar levels get much too low for the body to function normally.

If your symptoms suggest that you are perhaps a victim of this ailment, you have two routes to pursue. One is to have a physician review your history and send you to a lab for a glucose tolerance test lasting *at least five hours* with *at least seven blood samples.* The length of the test is very important, because a two-hour test will either appear normal or may show a hypoglycemic as a diabetic! Getting this test done is not as simple as it sounds because some physicians barely recognize this syndrome, or even that hypoglycemia exists. If you have difficulty in this regard, write to the Hypoglycemia Foundation, P.O. Box 98, Fleetwood, Mt. Vernon, N.Y. 10552, and request a list of physicians in your area who treat this ailment.

The second approach, if you feel you have the symptoms, is to realize that the medical treatment for the ailment is dietary, and you can put yourself on the same diet for some weeks. You will certainly notice a change in your mental, physical, and emotional condition if you are indeed hypoglycemic. You can obtain detailed dietary instructions from the Foundation listed above or from any of the references given later, but the general concept is a diet high in complete protein, moderate to high in fats (roughly half unsaturated), very low in simple sugars, and quite moderate in starches.

Recommended Foods: All lean meats, fish, poultry, shellfish, and eggs. All green leafy vegetables, tomatoes, cucumbers, squash, etc. Soybeans and soy products, nuts, seeds, and peanut butter. All fresh fruit, but citrus in moderation, canned or frozen fruit only if water-packed without sugar. Bread in moderate amounts, preferably whole wheat, rye, etc. Milk, cheese, and yogurt, excellent between meals or before bed.

Outlawed Foods: All sugars and honeys, and especially sugar-sweetened soft drinks. Sugar-sweetened juices, canned or frozen fruits. Vegetables packed in sugar-sweetened sauces or liquids. Potatoes, corn, rice, peas, lima beans, baked beans. Pasta, such as macaroni, spaghetti, etc. Pie, cake, pastries, candies, cookies, crackers, pretzels, potato chips, and all other sweet snack foods. Ice cream. Dates and raisins and other dried fruit. Cola drinks, coffee, and strong tea. All sweetened beverages. *All alcoholic beverages.*

Food intake should be distributed over six small meals a day, or three modest meals and three good-sized snacks. You should balance the size of portions to achieve the desired calorie level for your activities and weight. It is especially important to reduce your caffeine intake, as caffeine stimulates the adrenal glands, which in turn have a direct effect on the sugar production rate by the liver.

Perhaps it would be helpful to explain briefly the way sugar is handled in the body. When you eat starches or sugars, they are digested in the stomach (actually your saliva contains a very powerful enzyme for digesting starches, so they start to break down quickly) and are absorbed through the walls of the small intestine into the bloodstream. Regardless of the type of starch or complex sugar, they are absorbed as simple sugars, either glucose or fructose. In response to their presence in the blood, the pancreas releases insulin into the blood. When that insulin reaches the liver, it causes the liver to begin reducing the blood sugar level by converting the circulating sugars into glycogen, storing it for later use.

In the normal body, the circulating sugar level would be reduced to the normal level of 80 to 100 mg% (milligrams per 100 milliliters of blood). In the diabetic, it may stay as high as 300 to 400, and in the hypoglycemic, the liver may take the blood sugar level all the way down to 30 to 40, resulting in the symptoms we first described. This effect occurs especially when the body is confronted with a sudden massive infusion of sugar (How about a hot fudge sundae with a large soft drink?). If the food intake is scrambled eggs and a hamburger patty, the absorption is slower, and the protein is absorbed as amino acids. These are either used as such, or converted very slowly to glucose.

The adrenal glands can cause the liver to convert its stored glycogen back into blood sugar and, since the adrenals are stimulated by caffeine, coffee is normally to be avoided. In another part of this book, we mention the value of a cup of coffee at certain early stages of some headaches for its vasodilating ("vessel-dilating") effects. If you are hypoglycemic and wish to use this remedy in an emergency, please remember to eat some protein with your cup of coffee, perhaps some cheese or a handful of peanuts. It will make a world of difference.

Many, if not most, alcoholics are hypoglycemic, and since alcohol is metabolized just like a sugar, their problems are compounded. Generally they are vitamin deficient because of their poor dietary habits. The vitamin B complex and vitamin C are both very important to hypoglycemia, and you should consider using these supplements. The B complex is vital to sugar and carbohydrate metabolism in the human body, and deficiencies of these vitamins will result in metabolic abnormalities.

Vitamin C and the compounds called bioflavonoids, which occur naturally with it in citrus fruit, affect both blood vessel permeability and histamine levels. Histamine is released in muscle tension and allows the fluid carrier of the blood to seep through the walls of the capillaries, causing edema and swelling. Vitamin C both destroys histamine and alters the vessel wall permeability, so it may be very helpful in certain headache conditions.

There are very strong grounds to consider white sugar one of the most destructive ingredients to health in our entire environment. Consumption of sucrose by the American public has increased at radical rates, especially among children, with the introduction of the multiplicity of sweetened cereals, cakes, candies, and almost every prepackaged and preserved food. Anything you can do to decrease the total amount of sugar you consume is bound to be very constructive to your well-being, regardless of whether you are hypoglycemic. And if you *are* one of the many who suffer from this common but seldom-detected ailment, the results of adjusting your diet can be amazing.

Other Headaches

In this group are included headaches that seem to relate to some specific cause or sequence. They may also be tension or migraine headaches, but perhaps related to a more specific source. This section is written so that you will have some questions to address to your own headache history. If you are to cure your headaches, you want to be as familiar as possible with the potential triggers that initiate them.

The following brief descriptions may help you identify your syndrome. The important fact about all of these headaches, as well as migraines and tension headaches, is that the pain arises from the same sources in all cases: the blood vessels and musculature of the scalp, forehead, and neck. The system I recommend in this book will reduce the incidence of any and all of these types of headaches, and, if followed faithfully, will lead to *total freedom* from your headaches, regardless of the type.

Allergy Headaches: Since there are individuals who are allergic to almost any substance you can name, some only to one substance, and some allergic to many, this is a complex source. Be suspicious of your own headaches if they consistently have accompanying symptoms of running nose, weepy eyes, or sore throat, even if these are very mild effects. Keep an eye out also for links to specific locations, activities, or, most likely of all, a particular food or family of foods.

One of the common causes is tyramine, a substance found in cheddar and some other cheeses, most dairy products, beer, and some wines. Chocolate is the trigger for many. The so-called Chinese restaurant syndrome is brought on by monosodium glutamate (the notorious "MSG"), found in soy sauce and often used as a flavor enhancer. If you have a reaction to hot dogs, salami, bacon, and/or ham, you may be sensitive to the nitrites used as coloring agents in these foods. In examining your nutritional history, one tip is that some of us may be sensitive to a food at one time of the day, say at breakfast, but be able to eat it with impunity at any other time. So if you suspect this type of cause, keep a detailed diary for a few months; it may produce some real clues.

Sinus Headaches: The first thing to understand is that you probably don't have sinus headaches, because they are very rare. That sounds strange, in view of all the sinus medications sold in this country, but it is true. People with chronic sinusitis almost never suffer headaches from their sinus inflammation. This has been shown repeatedly in clinical studies, starting with the pioneering work of Dr. Wolff.

Acute sinus problems will sometimes lead to headaches, but

even these are not as common as most victims believe. The headache will usually come from muscle tension, perhaps related to the sinus victim's inactivity as the result of discomfort. Consequently, the treatment would be the same as for any other tension headache.

If you do feel you have a sinus headache, there are two very beneficial approaches. One is acupressure, using the pressure points for sinus as shown in chapter 5 together with the standard headache acupressure points. The second is heat, applied to the front of the face, both beneath and above the eyes. For some, the inhalation of warm, very moist air, as from a vaporizer, will also provide symptomatic relief. But keep in mind that in most cases, your headache is only indirectly related to the sinus congestion, and make use of my headache prevention emergency methods, as for any other headache.

Cluster Headaches: These are very violent headaches that strike in bursts over a few days or weeks, then may disappear for months or years. The victims are almost always rugged, very masculine-type men, frequently involved in hard or even dangerous work. Alcohol must be totally avoided when a cluster starts, as it is a very strong trigger for this type of attack.

Women's Headaches: These are almost certainly related to hormonal levels and are characterized by correlation with menstrual cycles, onset of menopause, etc. Several studies have shown that contraceptive pills produce frequent headaches in a significant proportion of women who were originally free of headaches. In addition, the pill will aggravate the condition of those with a migraine history.

Caffeine Withdrawal Headaches: Very heavy coffee drinkers (over six cups a day) must adjust their physiology to the continual stress to their adrenals, liver, and other organs, to the point that a sudden cessation of coffee intake can lead to severe headaches. The cure for this one is obvious, and I most certainly do *not* mean "to keep drinking coffee"! I *do* mean "taper off"!

Weekend Headaches: These may be so regular as to occur at almost exactly the same hour on Saturday or Sunday. Usually these are interpreted as signaling some family or husband-wife tension, such as a husband feeling guilty about scheduling his tennis or golf game at the very time he thinks he should be with his family. (These victims are usually male.) But another prime candidate is the "workaholic" (now beginning to include a growing number of career women) who really does feel guilty about doing anything other than working. In either case, try to understand that a proper amount of relaxation time is absolutely essential to your physical and emotional well-being, and to both your relationship to your family *and* your productivity in your work. If you have this problem, try altering your schedule in different ways. If your headache time is Saturday morning, try taking a few hours off during the week and working Saturday morning. Observe the effect, and adjust accordingly. Believe me, this is a problem you can work out with just a little creative thinking and the application of my system.

Hangover Headaches: This is a subject with which many of us have had some personal experience, but hangover headaches are not restricted to those of us with general headache tendencies. The most obvious way to avoid them is to not drink, but if that approach is too drastic, there are some steps you can take to minimize the aftereffects.

First, you should understand that the source is twofold: the alcohol itself, and the flavor and color elements in the liquor, known collectively as "congeners." Since these congeners arise from both the fermentation process and the aging process, they vary enormously with the type of liquor. They appear in greatest concentration and variety in those liquors we often refer to as "hard," i.e., bourbon, brandy, dark rum, and rye; are less concentrated in scotch and blended whiskies; and lowest in gin and especially vodka. This is some chemical support for the opinion that vodka produces less of a hangover effect than other liquors.

However, on top of the congener effects, there is the effect of the alcohol itself. It dilates the blood vessels, irritates the stomach, and interferes with water retention so that the body is dehydrated. The first step in protection (other than not drinking at all) is to slow down absorption by having food in the stomach before starting to drink. One of the most effective and convenient ways is to have a glass of milk beforehand.

After drinking, there are several steps that can be taken. It has been demonstrated that the ingestion of fructose, the fruit sugar, will increase the metabolism of alcohol by 15 to 30 percent, so a simple and effective remedy is to have a piece of toast liberally spread with honey before going to bed. An antacid to minimize stomach irritation is helpful. Because alcohol stimulates urine production, salts will be lost from the body, so drinking beef broth and/or vegetable juices the next morning will be constructive. Since position plays a role in hangover headache, taking a modest walk the next morning may considerably improve the slack and dilated blood vessels of the head.

Above all, one should *not* take another drink to relieve the hangover. This so-called cure is one of the sure signs of alcoholism!

Sexual Headaches: Regular attacks after intercourse identify this type, which in some cases is said to arise from guilt feelings or emotional frustrations associated with coitus.

Depression Headaches: Some clinical studies have shown that headache victims are more depressed than the norm, showing more psychosomatic pain, anxiety, and amnesia. No headache type has been shown to be consistently and strongly associated with any particular personality type. However, when the victim is chronically in a state of moderate depression, one might suspect what is called "vertebralbasilar insufficiency," or, more simply, an insufficient flow of blood to the brain stem areas. The basilar artery supplies blood to the brain stem, or lower part of the brain. This is part of the limbic system, which is related to an individual's mood. The arteries associated with the vertebrae can be compressed by bone spurs impinging upon the vertebral canal in the neck region (the so-called cervical vertebrae). Irritation of these arteries can produce sudden and strong headaches. An effect very similar to this is frequently found after "whiplash" injuries, which occur in car accidents where the head is thrust violently forward or back. In all of these cases, the relationship of headache and depression to mechanical alterations of the vertebrae themselves, either due to injury or degenerative disease such as arthritis, has been clearly shown. It strongly supports our general thesis that postural alignment, especially of the head, neck, and spine, is a vital factor in most headaches.

PART II

Curing Your Headache

The Magic Keys

My drugless system is based upon these four keys of headache prevention:

CIRCULATION
TENSION
TONE
POSTURE

Anyone who has headaches consistently, or who has extremely painful headaches, is below par in one or more of these elements.

The following chapters present a wide variety of methods for greatly improving each of the keys. Some of the techniques are required in my system of headache prevention; some techniques are left to your free choice. Your choice is dependent upon your individual circumstances, such as age, physical condition, life-style, work habits, and the relevance to your personal headache history.

Please read each chapter carefully and thoroughly. I have deliberately kept them quite brief to encourage your study. Even though a chapter may seem inappropriate, read it carefully. A point may come up that will have real impact. Remember, this is a "self-help" manual. I will prescribe certain specific methods that you must use every day, but examine the other material and select the specific methods of interest and relevance to you. Be open and willing to experiment. You know yourself better than anyone else does, so have confidence in your judgment. With your enthusiastic cooperation and my system, we should be able to eliminate your headaches.

CHAPTER 4

Holistic Medicine

Holistic Medicine, also referred to as "Integral Medicine" at some medical centers, is an ancient set of concepts that appears to be the wave of the future in American medicine. Simply stated, the central concept is that the human body is a "whole." Attempts to partition off the body into subsections, and to treat a single subsection as if it were unrelated to the rest of the body, are doomed to only partial success because of the intricate interrelations among all parts of the body.

If the front tires of your car were badly worn, but on the outer edges only, you would not simply buy new tires. You would be advised by the mechanic that the front end is out of alignment, and that you must have it realigned so you do not quickly ruin the new tires. Your body also needs frequent realignment and readjustment. A simple drug cannot do that. Holistic medicine starts with the assumption that in any ailment, the body must be treated as a whole. Modern medicine, while magnificent in its many achievements, has partially lost sight of the patient as a person, and sees the patient as a bag full of chemicals, to be tested by extracting a small sample by needle and running it through complex analyzers, to be treated by reinjecting some new chemicals back into the bag, either by needle or by mouth, and hoping that will cure all.

This is an approach that has been a smashing success for many virus diseases and almost all bacterial diseases. In fact, many of the most devastating diseases have been totally eliminated from the average American family. But modern medical practice has been depressingly unsuccessful with heart disease, arthritis, alcoholism, mental depression, drug abuse, certain forms of cancer, and *headaches*. A whole body approach to these problems is seen by many medical specialists as offering a better solution. Certainly a whole body approach can eliminate your tension and migraine headaches. *Your cure is within yourself.* We just have to help you dig it out.

The simplest examples of the holistic concept lie in the dietary field. Take the effect of vitamins, for example: if a young child has badly deformed legs from rickets, the problem actually lies in vitamin D deficiency in the diet, and that must be corrected before corrective measures can be taken on the obvious leg symptoms. In night blindness, it is not the eyes alone that are at fault, but a vitamin A deficiency in the entire body.

By now, we are all familiar with the effects the emotions can have on the body itself, but perhaps we are not willing to accept how strong that effect can be in ourselves. It is difficult to discuss this subject in depth without plunging into the complexities of human physiology and neuroanatomy, but let's give it a brief try. The key subject for us is the so-called autonomic nervous system. You might read that as the "automatic" nervous system, and immediately gain a good insight into what it is and does. The autonomic nervous system regulates and controls the activities of the body structures that are *not* under voluntary control and that, as a rule, function below the level of consciousness. Thus, breathing, blood circulation, the digestion of foods, body temperature, metabolism, sweating, and the secretion of certain endocrine glands are not under our normal control, but are regulated for us by the autonomic nervous system. To the headache victim, this system is especially important because of its control over the diameter of the blood vessels and hence of the blood flow through these vessels. This control is known technically as "vasoconstricting" or "vasodilating" ("vaso" meaning blood vessel, and "constricting" and "dilating" referring, of course, to either the shrinking or expanding of the diameter of the blood vessel). Although these systems are not thought to be under conscious control, it has long been recognized that outside stimuli can affect them. For example, when the body is heated, general vasodilation throughout the muscles occurs. There is a decrease in the vasoconstrictor tone as well as active vasodilation. Applied warmth in a local area causes vasodilation in parts remote from the point of application. Conversely, cold air on the bare back or arm causes vasoconstriction in the pharynx and nasal passages.

Deep breathing causes reflex constriction of the vessels of the skin, a slight fall in blood pressure, and a slowing of the peripheral blood flow. Generally, a painful stimulus will produce a vasoconstrictor response, plus an excitation of the psychic center and a release of adrenaline (the "fight or flight" response).

Many examples could be given, but the important point here is that your body, including the area where your headaches occur, is a complex of interacting systems. To eliminate a problem such as headaches, we will begin in the next chapter to utilize some approaches which initially may seem to you to be remotely related to your problem, but which, in fact, are highly and specifically relevant.

CHAPTER 5

Hands On

Brush It Away

This is probably the most important chapter in this book, and it deserves careful study. It provides a simple but unique method that anyone can use to solve one of the principal problems of all headache victims.

As we have shown in earlier chapters, the condition of the blood vessels and muscle tissue underlying the scalp is all-important in the prevention of headaches. The problem is to find a simple, quick, effective way to stimulate both the surface tissue *and* the underlying muscles and blood vessels, especially the arteries of the temples and back of the head. After much testing, I have devised a technique of massaging those areas with a specially selected brush, so that the patterned strokes not only stimulate the surface skin, but roll and push the underlying tissues, greatly improving the circulation through both the arteries and capillaries of the scalp muscles. This brings fresh oxygen to those tissues, and flushes metabolic waste products away, stimulating the growth of regular circulation through the scalp and neck.

The massage need not take very long, but it must be practiced *very consistently.* It must be done at least once a day, and the key areas, meaning temples, around ears, and back of head and upper neck, should be done two or three times a day, especially at the beginning of the program.

I will describe this massage procedure to you in detail, but first let me recommend strongly that you obtain the right kind of brush with which to do the massaging. It is possible to do it with the fingertips, but for maximum benefit it should be done with the brush for several reasons. It is much easier to deliver uniform pressure with the brush because it covers a much larger area than the fingertips. It is important to distribute the pressure evenly, because some parts of the underlying tissue are quite sensitive. Also, it is vital to get the scalp to move laterally and vertically over the underlying tissues. This can be done much more effectively with the brush because of its greater resistance against the skin as it is moved along. And last, but by no means least, the bristle tips of the brush provide a much-needed stimulation to the surface of the skin itself.

So get yourself a brush, preferably with a flat area of several square inches and a back shaped to fit the hand comfortably. Fortunately, there are many such brushes available, because the natural fiber bath brush (the type that usually has a long detachable handle, wooden back, and natural bristles) is sold in most department stores, health food stores, and bath shops. Other natural bristle brushes can be bought in variety stores, supermarkets, and discount drugstores, often sold as small inexpensive scrub brushes. The bristles should be fairly stiff but not as rigid as the typical hairbrush. An ideal bristle is the vegetable fiber often marked "Tampico." Synthetic bristles are less satisfactory because they tend to have sharp ends, which are too abrasive when moved across the skin.

If in doubt when selecting a brush, test it by massaging the back of your hand. Press the brush with moderate firmness against the back of your hand, and move it in small circles while gradually sliding it across the back of your hand. It should move the skin with it as you make the circles, but not cause skin abrasion as you move across. There should be a definite feeling of stimulation and very mild irritation but no pain. Generally, your scalp will be less sensitive than the back of your hand, so later you may wish to select a stiffer brush.

The next question is when to use the brush, and the answer is to make it an absolutely integral part of your toilet procedure morning and night. The whole massage takes less than ninety seconds, so time is not a problem for anyone; the problem is

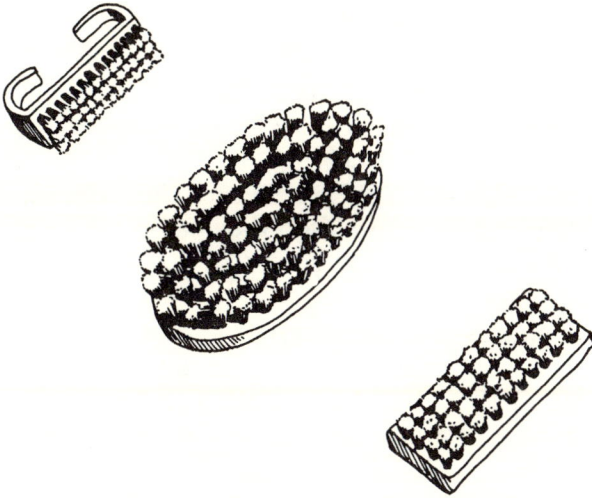

Center brush is best type; others are quite useable.

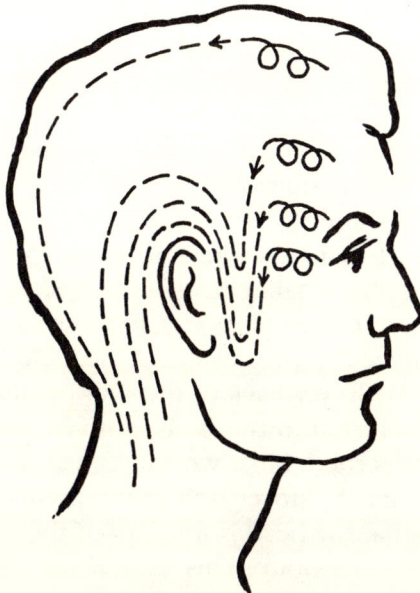

Brushing Pattern

remembering to do it consistently. So make it part of your regular routine twice a day. Since you clean your face morning and night, there is no better sequence than just before or after washing (or using your cleansing cream) to do the one-minute brush massage. This will do more than any other single thing you can do to normalize the muscle tone of the scalp and neck muscles and the tiny but all-important muscles of the blood vessel walls. After all, they are the muscles most directly related to your headaches (in fact, they cause your headaches), so it is a vital part of this program that they be afforded attention twice a day.

Remember, this entire program of headache prevention can take as little as ten minutes a day, so anyone can afford the time, but *no* part of that ten minutes is more important than this one minute of brush massage *each* morning and evening.

Now that we have selected your brush, and worked out your procedure for using it, let's discuss the way you will use it. The drawing shows the general pattern of the massage.

Starting at the intersection of the forehead and temple, just above the eyebrow, press the brush against the skin, and rotate it in small circles so that the upper part of the circle goes toward the back of your head. Feel good? Remember that on either side of the head, the brush makes its circle by being moved up-back-down-forward, in circles only about one-half inch in diameter. Study the drawing so that you understand the motion.

Now continue the small circles as you gradually move horizontally across the side of the head toward the ear. About midway between the eyebrow and ear, begin to descend toward the earlobe. At that point, reverse back up in front of the ear (still making the small circles in the same direction), pass above the ear as close to it as comfortable, and descend behind it, directly over the protrusion of your skull behind the ear. This area at the lower back of the skull, where large and small neck muscles attach to the skull, is a vital area as far as headaches are concerned. Most working positions (at a desk, typewriter, workbench, stove, sink, etc.) involve the torso tipped forward, so that the head is forward of the pelvis, or the head looking down, or both. This means the head is being supported by the neck muscles in a basically unbalanced position, with resultant stress on the skull area we have just reached with the brush massage. So this is a vitally important area. Massage it well, and move down into the trapezius, the sloping muscles at the back of your neck and shoulders.

Now go back to your starting point, but about one inch above the eyebrow, and repeat the same pattern, above the first pattern, but still dipping in front of the ear. Again, work well down the neck after paying good attention to the base of the skull.

And finally, for the third and last pass on this side, start over the eyebrow at your hairline, and repeat the same pattern toward the back of your head.

Now repeat the same sequence on the other side of your head, starting low on the head as before, working each pass higher. When finished with that side, start at your front hairline just to the right of the center of your head and do a series of circles back directly over the top of your head. Then do the same just to the left of the center of your head. At this point, some women may have problems with coiffures. If this is a problem when coupled with the morning rush to work, skip the overhead part on days when you need to, but be sure to include it on weekends, before shampoos, and at other times when you can squeeze it in.

Be sure to pay attention with careful brushing to the area just in front of the ear at the upper point of its attachment to the scalp. Through this area runs the main artery supplying the scalp, and it is also the point of insertion of the main chewing muscles of the jaw. Tension, of course, is often reflected in a clenching of the jaw, and it is at this point that the resultant congestion becomes most painful. We have already discussed the importance of this artery and the temporal branch of the facial artery, which also goes through this same area. This potential hotbed of trouble is a key area for attention during brush massage. In fact, this and the lower back of the head (the occipital area) are the two parts that need the most consistent massage; if, during the day, you feel any signs of tension building up, or a hint of a headache coming on, use your fingers for an immediate brief massage of these points. If you feel you need deeper massage, use the thumbs. For the side of the head, place the fingers together on the forehead and the thumbs will fall naturally into place, as well as having a base against which to control the pressure. For the lower back of the head, place the knuckles directly over your ears, and again the thumbs will be in the proper places. In both cases, the massage should be done with a small, rolling motion and enough pressure to move the underlying muscle tissue.

The whole brush massage procedure discussed above need take no longer than one and a half minutes. This adds up to only three minutes per day, a small enough time commitment for the enormous benefits to be derived. I cannot over emphasize how crucial this brush massage is to my approach to eliminating headaches. In addition, it is a great wakeup tool in the mornings, and a wonderful relaxer at bedtime. Odd, that it can act both ways, but, like any massage, the effects can be enormously varied by rate, intensity, and duration, all of which are under your personal control.

Some of you may wonder why this simple brush massage can be so extremely effective. The answer is that same old word we worked over earlier: *circulation.* It is almost overobvious to state that "blood is the lifeblood of the tissues," but think about that for a moment. It not only supplies the oxygen vital to normal respiration of the cells, but removes the waste products of metabolism such as lactic acid. We are all familiar with the fatigue and soreness that develop in large muscles of the arms, legs, or back after vigorous exercise or work. We are also familiar with the typical relief procedures, such as soaking in a hot tub, massage, sweating in a steam bath or sauna, or using an electrical heating pad. What do all these methods do? They *increase* circulation. The stiffness is a result of metabolic end products that are still lodged in the large muscle tissues, and the only way to remove them is for increased circulation to sweep them away to the liver and other tissues where the metabolism can be completed.

As I say, we are all familiar with and accept the above, yet we seem unaware of the fact that on a small (but oh, so important) scale this happens in the muscles of the scalp and neck. When some of these muscles remain contracted for too long, whether from position or from nervous tension, circulation is decreased in the muscles at the same time that metabolic products are building up, resulting in the "worst of both worlds." Alternating contractions and relaxations in a muscle are a great aid to circulation.

It may be helpful to digress for a moment to consider the way the thigh muscles, sometimes referred to as the "second heart," contribute to circulation during walking. When the thigh muscles relax, the arterial blood rushes down the leg, propelled both by the heart and by gravity. That flow also pushes the venous blood up into the veins of the leg, against gravity. When the thigh muscles contract, they squeeze on the veins, propelling the venous blood on up toward the heart. All muscle groups act this way on the veins passing through them. If you don't believe it is important, try the simple test of standing in a half-crouch without moving for a short time. The leg muscles, which can carry us easily for hours when walking, complain after less than a minute if shortened to a fixed degree and not allowed to move.

I hope the analogy is obvious. If you are going to lean over a desk or table or sink for some period of time, keep moving and flexing, even if almost imperceptibly, or small cramps will begin. If a major cramp occurs it produces pain, and you are immediately aware of it; you move, squeeze the offending muscle or shake it out, and, unless it is a severe "charley horse," all is generally well in a few minutes. But if only small parts of the muscle are involved initially, no pain appears, you are not alerted, and you continue to inflict punishment on the muscle. Maybe not right away, but soon, you will pay the price: Headache.

If you massage those muscle areas properly, the circulation removes the offending metabolic products, and no buildup occurs. I know this sounds like a very simple solution to a frightening problem, but it works!

Alternative to Brushing

There will be times when your brush will not be available. Perhaps you are on a trip and forgot to pack it, or you are out to dinner and the telltale symptoms of an imminent headache begin their invasion. You don't have your brush, but don't panic. There is a way to get by with your bare hands!

The pattern of stimulation is just like you use with the brush. Start at the corners of the eyes, back toward the ears, down in front of the ears, up and over the ears, and on down to that key projection at the back of the skull. But now it must be done in two sequences: first with the fingertips, and then in a different fashion with the edges of the fingernails.

First, the use of the fingertips. There are two basic hand positions, either with the heels of the hands against the jaw or with the hands fully in the air, although at the same height. This is a matter of personal preference, although the freehand approach gives greater flow to the massage. In this first phase, only the fingertips should contact the skin, *not the fingernails.* The motion is rotary, as with the brush, but the pressure level against the skin is important. The fingers must press on the skin firmly enough so that as the fingers make their small circles, the skin moves freely over the underlying tissue, but without creating a feeling of great pressure against the underlying muscles. The pattern of circles should continue as with the brush, with particular attention paid to the temples, in front of the ears, and the back of the skull and down the neck. After the third pass, continue down the large muscle at the back of the neck (the trapezius) down into the shoulder. At this point, the rotary motion can evolve into a deep muscle massage, with the full hand grasping the bulk of the muscle and squeezing strongly as the fingers slide up over the top of the muscle.

Now repeat the sequence, closing the hand slightly so that the fingernails are perpendicular to the skin and the tips of the nails rest directly against the skin. Instead of a rotary movement, the hands oscillate from front to back so that the edges of the nails of all four fingers slide back and forth on the scalp. Be sure the motion is horizontal to start with, not up and down. The pressure should be modest, producing a tingling sensation but no real irritation.

As your hands move back toward the ears, elevate your elbows; your hands will rotate so that the nails can slide up and down in front of the ears, an important place when treating incipient headaches. Now work the hands back up to the tops of the ears, drop the elbows, and vibrate above the ears. Again the elbows come up, and the vibration is carried down behind the ears to the *most important spot:* the occipital protuberance (the bony lumps) behind the ears. This is a key area in the tension of headaches, whether it is the source of the tension causing the ache itself, or whether it is tension arising from the pain in an adjacent area. So go over these lumps thoroughly. Often a headache can be completely stalled if the vicious cycle of tension can be broken at this point.

The beauty of this technique is that it can be done in a few minutes with just your hands. If the signs of an impending headache appear at an important meeting or at a large family dinner, excuse yourself, retire to the nearest bathroom or rest-room, and do a sixty-to-ninety-second fingertip and nail massage. It will positively break up the progress of the pain, and no one will even suspect your problem. Women will find that, with a little practice, the entire sequence can be performed without disrupting their hairstyles.

The confinement and lack of motion on long airplane flights can often lead to tension in the neck and shoulders, and this can easily lead to a headache. By applying this method one hand at a time, you can ward off a headache without your fellow passengers ever noticing your self-treatment.

Trapezius Massage

The trapezius muscle may be the most important muscle in the body, as far as headaches are concerned. The trapezius is the large muscle at the back of the neck. It is really two muscles, one on each side, each triangular in shape, with the long side of the triangle running vertically along the spine, one point at the bony lumps at the rear of the head, the other point halfway down the back. The third point of the triangle is out behind the shoulder.

A primary function of this muscle is to hold the head erect, and that is why it is so involved in the headache sequence we are discussing in this book. To reiterate: almost every work or hobby function that we perform involves tipping the head forward; desk work, typing, reading in general, even much skilled labor, *all* involve looking down and, therefore, tipping the head forward. In this position, the head is supported by the trapezius muscle.

Muscles are at their best when rhythmically contracting and extending; that's why we can walk for long periods of time without much fatigue in the large muscles of the legs—they are alternating their motions beautifully, and in that process pumping freshly oxygenated blood into their capillaries. When you tire while walking, you will usually feel the fatigue in some part of the back and shoulders, indicating that you are walking well with the lower part of your body, but are not getting the same kind of fluid continuity in the upper part. In other words, you are constraining the motion in the back and shoulders, holding these parts in a rigid or semirigid fashion so

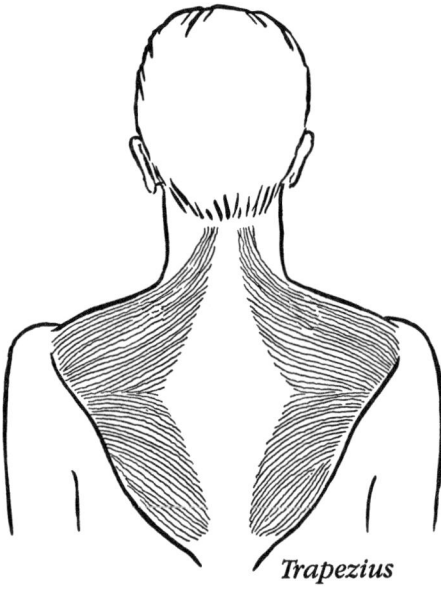

Trapezius

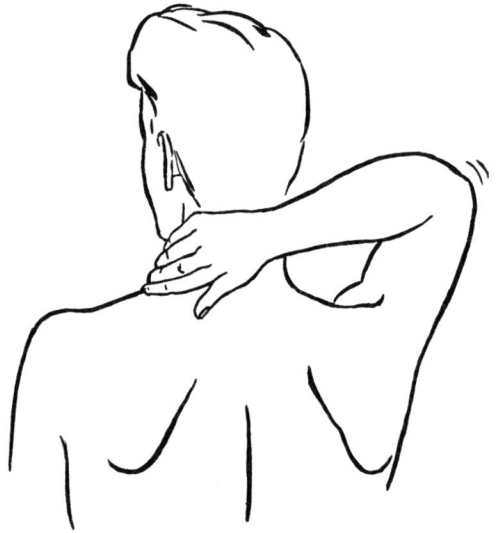

Behind the Neck Massage

that the muscle is not alternately contracting and extending, but is staying in a continuously contracted state. This is *terrible* for circulation in that muscle.

You must keep the muscle tissue open enough that blood can freely flow through, supplying oxygen and removing lactic acid and other waste products.

Although the trapezius can be literally a "pain in the neck," one advantage of its location is that you have good access to the most important part with your own hands. Why? For massage. If the problem were in the lower back, a sacroiliac problem needing massage, that means another person must do it, because it is out of your reach. But the part of the trapezius most likely to give trouble is the upper part and, if properly approached, this is well within your own massage range.

There are two basic kinds of massage: light or surface, and deep muscle. Light massage is used to stimulate the skin and underlying tissues and increase peripheral circulation. Deep massage is done to break up muscle congestion. In the pre-headache muscular strain phase, both kinds of massage are usually needed.

There are two prime areas for massage of the trapezius, one directly behind the neck, the other on top of the shoulders as they slope away from the neck.

Behind the Neck: Whether sitting or standing, be sure to be in an erect position with the chest up and the head slightly back. The key is to have the head far enough back so that the trapezius is not supporting the head, and is therefore loose. Place your hand on the back of your neck, squeezing slightly, and then incline your head forward and backward. You can easily feel when the muscle is tense and when it is relaxed. To perform the massage, place one hand on the back of your neck, lift the elbow of that arm until it is above the shoulder and pointed away from the body at about a 45° angle. Note: do not pull the elbow back too far or you will contract another part of the trapezius too strongly. Place the side of your thumb against the large vertebrae at the base of the neck (the third cervical, if you will), and let the heel of the hand press firmly into the neck so that it is almost wedged between the skull (just under and behind the ear) and the intersection of the neck and shoulder.

When you have placed it properly, and have allowed your

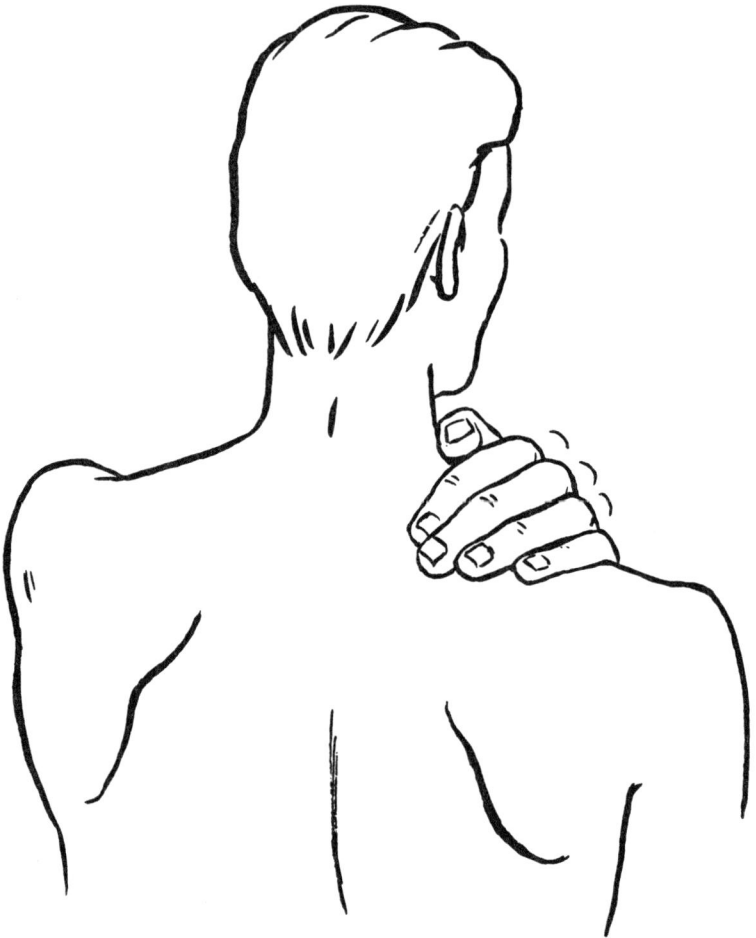

Top of the Shoulder Massage

head to tip back slightly, you will find a position where there is literally a "handful" of muscle that can be strongly kneaded by the fingers curling in toward the neck. Dig your fingertips into these muscles, then squeeze them toward your palm, allowing the fingertips to roll over the surface of the muscles while digging in strongly. Shift the hand slightly up and down so that the area from just under the skull all the way down into the upper shoulder can be kneaded. Be sure that the nonworking arm is supported in the lap or on the arm of a chair so that it is not being held up by the other trapezius. As your working hand grips down into the area at the base of the neck, you can tell immediately whether it is loose. If not, shift your arm and shoulder until it is really free.

Now repeat with the other hand, on the other side of your neck. The specific procedure is to do about five or six squeezes on one side, working down from the skull toward the shoulder, then reverse hands and repeat the process. Alternate sides and do each two or three times. Do not spend too long on one side, or you risk increasing tension in the other side from the elevated arm.

Top of the Shoulder: Again the opposite hand is used. Place the heel of the hand above the collarbone so that the fingers can extend well down the back. Start at the outer edge of the shoulder and work in toward the neck, reaching down past the upper edge of the shoulder blade and digging in the fingertips as if to roll the muscle tissue up toward the shoulder line. Work across the back until you feel the spine, then switch to the other hand and do the other side. As above, use about five or six deep squeezes to a side, then change, and repeat two or three times.

In both sequences, you are likely to find certain areas that are very sensitive, even quite painful, to your squeeze. *Good!* That confirms the diagnosis of muscular congestion, perhaps even a cramp, and delineates the real need for this massage. As with other procedures we have outlined, this can be done in only a minute, almost anywhere, without disrupting your normal routines in any way. But do it at the first signs of tension always; do not wait until it has become really worrisome.

When done properly, this relieves neck tension so completely that it can become addictive.

Face and Scalp Calisthenics

These movements should be done daily in front of your mirror. They will relax and tone the muscles of the face and scalp, not only helping your headache problems, but also improving your appearance. Most important, you will be relearning conscious control over these muscles and increasing the range through which you can move them. This is vital to this program because these movements are a simple and effective way to relax the scalp muscles when you feel tension starting to build or sense any sign of an impending headache. *Do each three times.*

1. *Eyebrows up and return:* Lift both eyebrows up quickly, as in surprise, with a strong tension at the top. Then relax and let them drop back down.

2. *Right eyebrow up and return:* Some of you may have difficulty at first in doing one brow. If so, start by holding the other in place with a forefinger and you will quickly catch on to the sensation. Again, pull strongly upward.

3. *Left eyebrow up and return.*

4. *Squint both eyes closed and release:* Squeeze both eyes into an exaggerated squint by rolling up both cheeks as much as possible until your eyes are squeezed tightly closed. Squint quickly, hold briefly, and relax.

5. *Squint right eye and release:* Squeeze right side of face hard enough to pull up corner of mouth.

6. *Squint left eye and release.*

7. *Frown deeply and release:* Squeeze brows both down over eyes and in toward bridge of nose.

8. *Wiggle ears or scalp above ears:* Some people can remember the childhood talent of wiggling their ears. But, if not, you can learn to activate the muscles under the scalp above and behind the ears. To start, place your hands loosely over your ears with the fingers bent and separated so that the fingertips rest against the scalp lightly. They should cover an arc from just above the front of the ear to the bony protuberances behind the ear. Now try to move this part of the scalp or your ears and you will feel small motions under your fingertips. Feel how you can increase or change this motion, and you will soon be moving this part of your scalp easily. This is a vital area for the prevention of both tension and migraine headaches, so some faithful practice at this movement will really pay off.

9. *Yawn wide and close:* Open the mouth by lowering the jaw slowly to as wide a position as is comfortable. Do not move very quickly and do not strain. Then close slowly.

10. *Open jaw, move right and left:* Open mouth slightly and then slide jaw from right to left and back.

11. *Wrinkle nose:* Squeeze nose up toward bridge as if smelling a really bad odor.

12. *Make faces:* This is an ad-lib; make like a kid and screw your face all around, moving brows, forehead, nose, mouth, jaw, and cheeks back and forth to get everything loose and moving. Enjoy it!

These are great to do while driving a car (except #4, of course), but when you stop for a traffic light you may find the driver of the car in the next lane giving you some very strange glances.

Face and Scalp Calisthenics (Three Repetitions Each)

1. Eyebrows up and return
2. Right eyebrow up and return
3. Left eyebrow up and return
4. Squint both eyes closed and release
5. Squint right eye and release
6. Squint left eye and release
7. Frown deeply and release
8. Wiggle ears or scalp above ears
9. Yawn wide and close
10. Open jaw, move right and left
11. Wrinkle nose
12. Make faces!

Neck and Shoulder Rejuvenators

All of these movements should be done *every day* in a quiet, relaxed manner, except the last two, which are more vigorous. These are not exercises for muscle development, but relaxing rejuvenators, designed to loosen the muscles, normalize the muscle tone, and increase your kinesthetic sense (that is, put you more in touch with the individual muscles). The latter is important not only for these motions themselves, but for use during your alpha sessions, so that you can "speak" directly to the muscles you wish to influence. *Each motion should be done three times,* with a slight pause at each flex point, and a definite pause at each return point. Start out doing them in front of a mirror. If you cannot do them that way all the time, check yourself at least once a week. Be conscious of your posture; stand tall (but not stiff!) when starting each movement. Think of the top of your head being suspended from the ceiling. Tuck in your pelvis, lift up your rib cage, and breathe naturally.

1. *Both shoulders raise and return:* With arms hanging loosely at your sides, lift both shoulders toward your ears. Do not squeeze too tightly; simply raise your shoulders fairly quickly, pause slightly, and lower all the way, with a full relaxation of the trapezius.

2. *Both shoulders circle forward:* Press shoulders back, then up, forward, and down, so that they make a complete circle in the air. For pace, try saying slowly, "one thousand one, one thousand two, one thousand three," completing one circle with each phrase.

3. *Both shoulders circle backward:* Just the reverse of above; move shoulders forward, then up, back, and down. In both #2 and #3, try to make as large a circle as possible without straining.

4. *Right shoulder up and return:* Just like #1, but single shoulder.

5. *Left shoulder up and return.*

6. *Right shoulder circle forward:* Same as #2, but one side.

7. *Left shoulder circle forward.*

8. *Right shoulder circle backward:* Same as #3, but one side.

9. *Left shoulder circle backward.*

10. *Rotate head right and return:* With head tall and level (check in mirror), turn head to right, keeping level, pause slightly, and return. With time, try to gradually increase amount of rotation *(no forcing).*

11. *Rotate head left and return.*

12. *Tilt head right and return:* Simply incline ear toward right shoulder, pause slightly, and return. Check in mirror to be sure that your head does not rotate left or right, but continues to face directly forward as it tilts. Do this one carefully and do

not strain. Initially your motion may be quite limited, but it will slowly increase.

13. *Tilt head left and return.*

14. *Chin toward chest and return:* From starting position, lower chin by tilting head forward on your neck; do not allow the whole neck and head to slump forward. You can check this by placing your fingers on the front of your throat. Your chin should squeeze down on these fingers if the movement is done properly.

15. *Chin toward ceiling and return:* Don't let the neck collapse, but keep the neck tall and point chin up toward the ceiling.

16. *Head circle right:* Start as in #15, then from chin-high position roll your head slowly to just above the right shoulder, through chin-down position, across above the left shoulder and back to chin-up position. Try to make a nice smooth motion, no snapping, and not too wide a circle at first. It will widen by itself as you loosen up.

17. *Head circle left:* Do not be surprised if you have more trouble going in one direction than the other. Most of us are unsymmetrical in terms of muscle tensions, and this is reflected in our movements.

18. *Neck stretch forward and back:* Keeping the chin level, move face forward toward the mirror as far as is comfortable, then move face back as far as possible with chin still level. Stop at center for a short pause before starting the next repetition. (Feel like a chicken?)

19. *Shoulder stretch:* Without raising your shoulders, extend your arms out to each side. Now push arms out to maximum reach, pause slightly, and, keeping arms level, shorten your reach by retracting the shoulder blades toward the backbone. Your shoulders may roll slightly forward and back as they move in and out, and that is fine. This is not a large movement, but *so* beneficial.

20. *Upright back stroke:* Now move to a place where you have plenty of room, stand tall, and alternately swing each arm in a circle, up in front, overhead, down in back, like swimming the back stroke, except not bending at the elbows. Start with five repetitions of right-left, right-left, etc., so that your arms follow each other around smoothly. Work up to ten repetitions, trying to get a good loose shoulder motion into the swing. (Don't drop your head forward.)

21. *Bend forward swimming stroke:* This is one of the absolutely best neck, shoulder, and back looseners. Place one foot slightly ahead of the other (right foot in front one day, left foot in front the next). Now bend forward from the waist, flexing your knees, so that your back is almost parallel to the floor. Look at the floor, keep your head fairly still, and *swim!* Bring your arm up with a bent elbow, the elbow quite high, then reach way forward with your hand, pointing fingers, and pull hand and arm back through the "water," bending the elbow slightly. Carry through until hand is behind hip, then lift up and over again, alternating arms. Get your shoulders to roll freely with each stroke so the whole upper back flexes. Work up to ten repetitions.

22. *Deep breathe:* Stand tall, relax, and take three deep breaths.

Neck and Shoulder Rejuvenators
(Three Repetitions Each, Except #20 and #21)

1. Both shoulders raise and return
2. Both shoulders circle forward
3. Both shoulders circle backward
4. Right shoulder up and return
5. Left shoulder up and return
6. Right shoulder circle forward
7. Left shoulder circle forward
8. Right shoulder circle backward
9. Left shoulder circle backward
10. Rotate head right and return
11. Rotate head left and return
12. Tilt head right and return
13. Tilt head left and return
14. Chin toward chest and return
15. Chin toward ceiling and return
16. Head circle right
17. Head circle left
18. Neck stretch forward and back
19. Shoulder stretch
20. Upright back stroke
21. Bend forward swimming stroke
22. Deep breathe

Acupressure

Although acupuncture and its finger-pressure variations have been in use in the Far East for thousands of years, the subject burst upon the West a few years ago as new relations with the People's Republic of China permitted a number of well-respected western physicians to observe the clinical use of these techniques. As usual with our news media, attention was directed primarily to the more startling applications, such as major abdominal surgery with no anesthesia other than that produced by a few small metal needles inserted at key points.

The witnesses were too authoritative to simply shrug off, so medical science began to take a closer look at this phenomenon. And, lo and behold, it turned out to be real: it has now been reliably established that there are indeed lines or series of points along various parts of the body (called "meridians" by acupuncturists) which have unusual properties and which interact with other parts of the body.

For example, the electrical resistance of the skin can be measured quite accurately with modern instruments. Although it will vary with perspiration and other factors, normal dry skin will show a surface resistance of about 500,000 ohms. But as the skin is tested point by point, one comes to certain small areas where the resistance will be only 12-15,000 ohms. When these points are marked, they turn out to be the traditional acupuncture points and meridians. Stimulation of these points produces effects at other points along the meridians. In some cases, central body effects are also produced.

Western theoretical explanations for these points and meridians are less well developed at this time than the physical proof of their existence. A noted Russian physicist has proposed that they represent an entirely separate circulatory system in which some form of energy (the Chinese call it *chi*) flows throughout the body. Other scientists have proposed explanations dealing with the interaction of the stimulation (whether by needle, pressure, or massage) of the known nerve structures of the body with the lower, more central parts of the brain, which are more ancient in terms of genetic development.

Regardless of explanations, the facts are now clear that acupuncture works, and many of the pain clinics at major medical centers in this country now use acupuncture, in various forms, as part of their normal treatment routine. Fortunately, you do not need to use the actual needles to benefit from this method. Finger-pressure methods have also been in existence for centuries, perhaps predating the needle technique. They have appeared in several variations, such as "acupressure," "Dō-in," and "Shiatsu." Each of these has some minor variations as to how the finger pressure is delivered, but all use the same "points" for the delivery of the pressure and, in general, agree on the locations relating to particular complaints or ailments. The exact method of applying the stimulation does not appear to be critical to success. The points involved with headache treatment may often be quite tender initially, so start with care and a soft touch, no more than twice a day, unless a critical headache situation arises.

The beauty of this technique lies also in the fact that you can do it on yourself, at any time, and in almost any situation. Because you are treating yourself, choose whichever thumb or fingertip can be most easily applied to the point of interest. Some methods use steady pressure, some use a squeeze-and-relax alternation, and some use a small rotation or vibration of the pressing finger or thumb. You may use any or all of these, guided by the feelings and sensations you obtain. As I said above, many of the points may be tender at times. Some are nearer the skin surface, while others lie deeper. On some of the leg and foot points, you may feel a paresthesia. This is the medical term for the sensation of hitting your "crazy bone" at the elbow, and deep pressure on some of the points will produce a tingling sensation shooting out from the point. Do not press so hard that real pain is produced; that is not conducive to healing. The pressure should be applied for twenty to thirty seconds, but the actual time is not critical. Since the points are in pairs, on both right and left sides of the body, remember to treat *both* sides. If you have trouble locating any of the points, remember to feel for the tenderness or the slight "crazy bone" feeling, and that will be the point.

Use of these points on a daily basis will normalize or "tune up" the nervous system and body as a whole, but in the headache syndrome, which is our main concern, the chief advantage is the ability to apply acupressure the minute the first symptoms of a headache appear, and totally stop its development. Learn the key acupressure points by heart. There are not many, and you will then be prepared to use them at those vital times when only *you* know how much dreaded discomfort and pain you are preventing.

You should, however, understand one qualification about the use of acupressure. It will not prevent the *starting* of headache symptoms. It will stop the discomfort once the headache has started, but to eliminate the problem of headaches starting, you must use my entire system consistently. Except for the "tune-up" points, acupressure simply modifies the symptoms. It will not eliminate the root cause, but it is a fantastic emergency treatment.

Acupressure Points

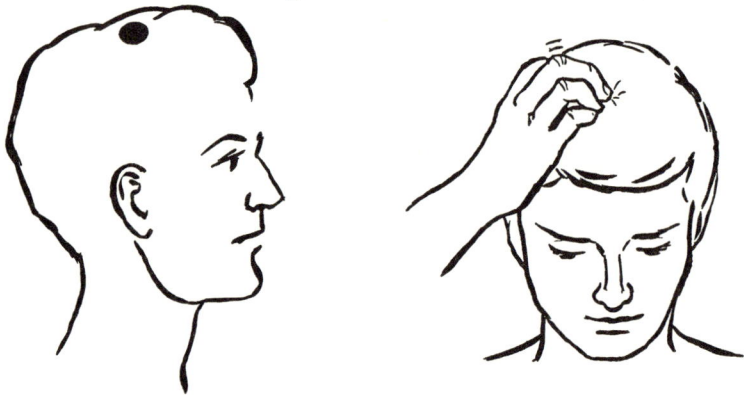

Top of Head: *Directly on top of the head, in the middle of a line connecting the tops of the ears. Use second finger to press strongly with rotation.*

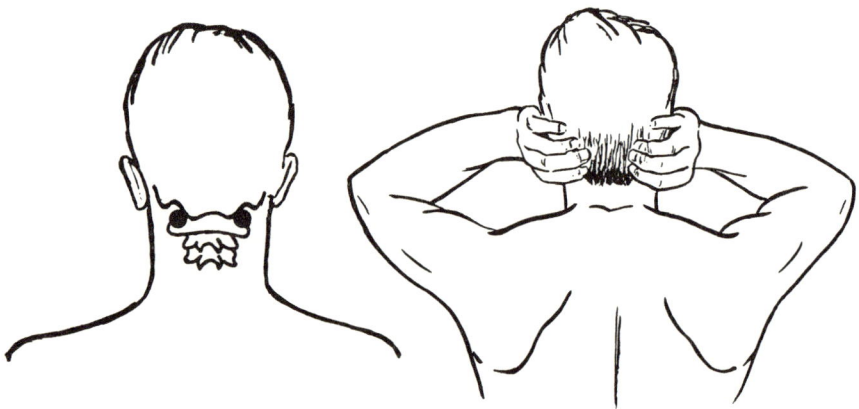

Back of Head: *Feel the back of your head, about the level with the earlobe, for two "bumps," one on each side of the midline. Then lower your fingers about an inch until you are under the bumps. Rock your head slightly back until you feel the neck muscles relax. You can either bring your elbows forward and massage with your fingertips, or pull your elbows back and massage with your thumbs. Use whichever position permits you to apply strong pressure.*

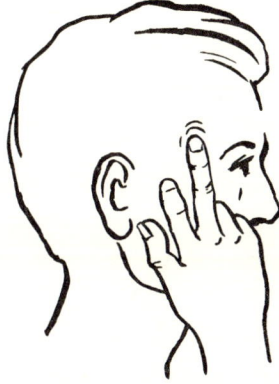

Side of Head: *Temple: Behind eyebrow, at same level, feel for depression in skull. Rotate end of middle finger, and remember both sides.*

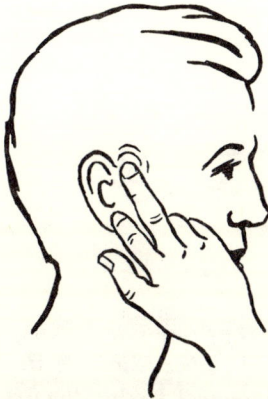

Front of Ear: *Feel for depression in front of upper earlobe, in front of jaw muscle attachment.*

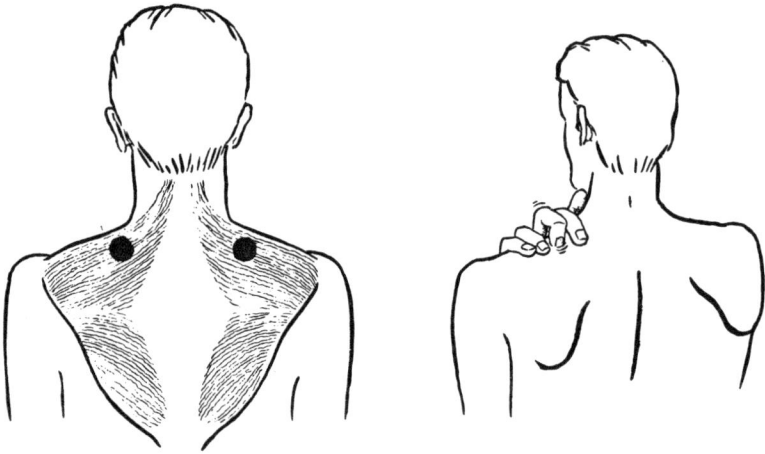

Shoulder: *Place heel of right hand on your left collarbone, so that your thumb is against your neck, and your fingers drape over your shoulder. The tip of your middle finger will now rest over the acupressure point and should be dug in forcefully while wiggling it up and down rapidly.*

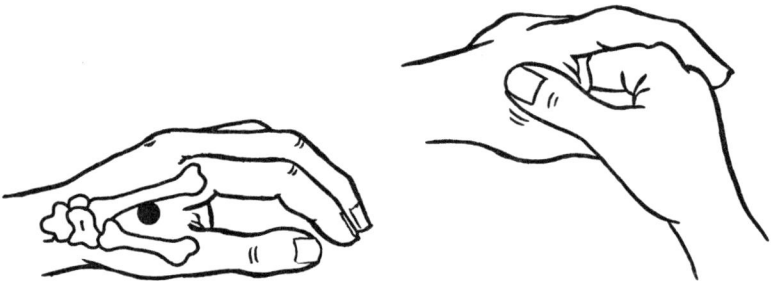

Hand: *Open thumb of one hand, with fingers flat, until the web between thumb and index finger is stretched slightly. Then place opposite thumb on the web so that the first joint is on the edge of the web. The tip of the thumb will now be against the acupressure point, on the bone going to the index finger. Remember to reverse and do both hands each time you use this one.*

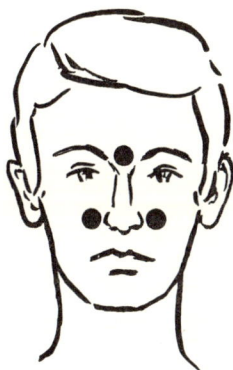

Sinus: *Between eyebrows; on each side of nose. Massage firmly with end of finger.*

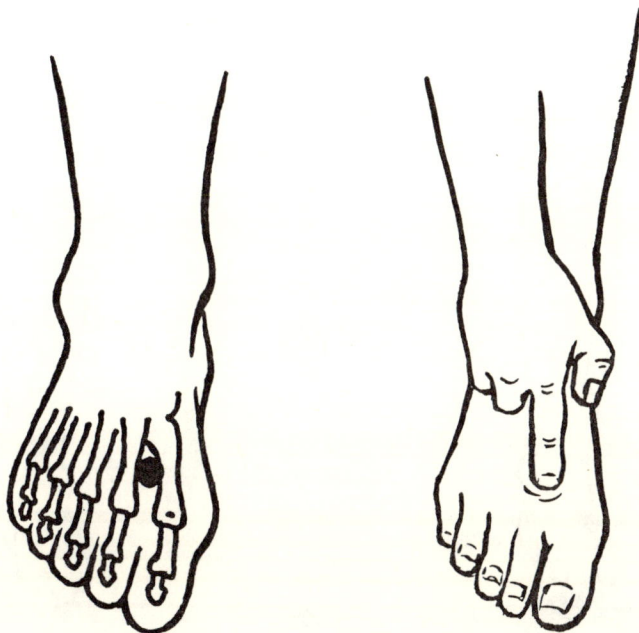

Top of Foot: *On the top of the foot, in the depression between the first and second toes, about an inch above the web between the toes.*

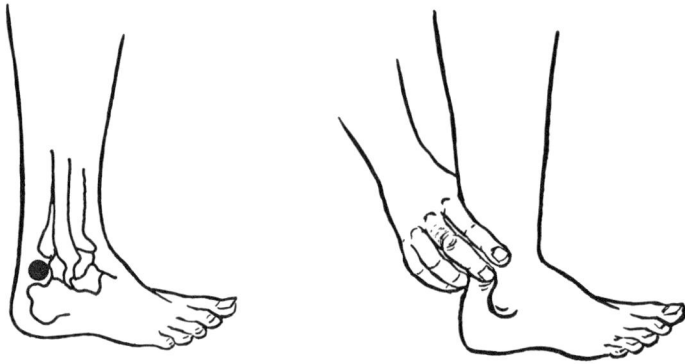

Achilles Tendon: *This point is on the outside of the ankle, behind the ankle bone and just in front of the Achilles tendon of the heel. One way to get good pressure on this point is to place your arm inside your leg while sitting, so that your elbow is against your inner thigh. Your fingers will just reach the point comfortably, and the arm against your leg will allow you good leverage for firm pressure with the tip of the second finger.*

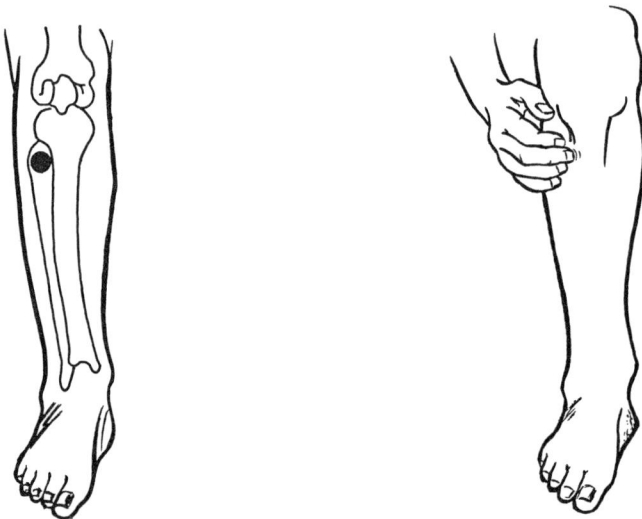

Shin: *Place second finger of right hand on right kneecap. Now slide down to the next lump, which is the head of the tibia (the shinbone). Slide to the outside of the shinbone, and down about an inch. You will find a spot that is sensitive when you press in against the side of the shinbone; that is your spot. Remember to do both legs.*

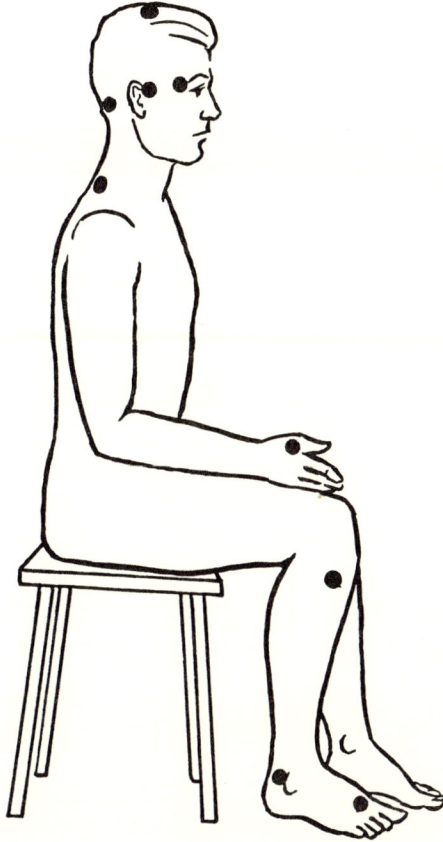

Summary of Headache Acupressure Points: *Please practice and* memorize.

CHAPTER 6

Shape Up

Posture

Since you are interested in preventing any more headaches, you must be interested in your posture. It has been clearly shown that muscle tension is involved in, and is often the start of, the vast majority of headaches, and posture is a major factor in muscle tension.

The term "muscle tension" is used to describe that situation in which muscles are consistently overcontracted. If you lift a heavy book from a table with one arm, naturally your biceps muscle will contract, to resist the weight or to bend the arm at the elbow. That is not "muscle tension." As you lay the book back down, the biceps relaxes and lengthens again. Muscles come in pairs; one is extended as the other contracts. For example, the biceps, on the front of the upper arm, bends the arm at the elbow. The triceps, on the back of the arm, straightens the arm at the elbow. Normally, a muscle contraction results in movement.

But now suppose you want to "make a muscle" in your biceps, as small boys or body-builders are apt to do. You don't want your elbow to flex so much that your hand is up against your shoulder, so you contract not only the biceps but also the opposing triceps (feel the back of your arm). Thus, no movement occurs, although both muscles may be in maximum contraction. This is an extreme version of "muscle tension."

Muscle has a quality called "tone." The word is used by athletes, dancers, physiologists, physicians, and others to refer to an ill-defined quality that muscle tissue has in the relaxed state of normal posture. The body has a bony skeleton, of course, but since that skeleton is beautifully jointed, we would fall over in a heap if our muscles were to totally relax. Normal muscle tone keeps the body in the desired position, with no conscious effort on our part. Too low muscle tone results in the flabby, drooping musculature that we normally associate with the unathletic or older body (although in this day and age of the eternal automobile, we see it more and more in even the teenage body). Too high muscle tone results in the tight, tense musculature we associate with the neurotic, compulsive individual; in other words, a great deal of muscle tension.

The state of contraction of the body muscles is obviously affected by the load put on them, and this is where posture enters the picture. As poor posture forces the body out of alignment, and consequently out of balance, the muscles have to contract in abnormal ways, often remaining contracted for hours on end. The most obvious culprit is, of course, the head. Not only is it heavy (about 10 percent of the body weight), but the head can get strong leverage on those neck and back muscles, making them work very hard. This creates muscle tension. Obviously, muscle tension can also arise from nervous tension, but as we treat that in another chapter, let's take a hard look now at posture. But instead of starting with the head, we'll start with the real core of posture, the pelvis.

The pelvis is the center of the body, even more so than the waist. It is where the largest, most flexible hinges of the body are located—the hip joints. The pelvis is the key to walking, standing, and sitting. The epitome of good posture lies almost halfway between the slump that most of us fall into, especially when tired, and the academy-cadet military erectness that many of us affect when told to "stand up straight." These extremes are both equally unhealthy.

Good posture starts with an acceptance of the fact that the spine normally has slight curvatures at several points and cannot really be made straight. These curves must not be exaggerated, however. Since you cannot see your spine directly, you must observe the curvatures indirectly, by sensing the positions of the pelvis, chest, shoulders, neck, and head. When standing or walking, knees and feet must also be considered.

Sitting is what most of us do most of the time, so we will start with that position. The pelvis contains the bones upon which we sit, or upon which we *should* sit. To observe a teen-age movie audience, one would think that we were designed to sit upon our lower backs! In youth, of course, one's body can take all kinds of punishment with little obvious effect other than the creation of bad habits.

Good sitting posture starts with the small of the back firmly against the back of the chair, feet on the floor, the body weight firmly on top of the pelvis. Be careful, though, not to tilt the pelvis forward so that the small of the back pulls away from the chair. Consider that the head, torso, and pelvis form one vertical line, with the pressure of your body weight being felt clearly directly on your seat, not high up on the buttocks. If in doubt, slip your hand under your seat and feel the down-pointing ends of your pelvis that constitute your sitting bones. Balance on those bones so that your weight is directly over them.

Now balance your chest and head so that they are directly over those sitting bones. A vertical line dropped down through the top of your head should go down through the middle of your shoulders, the center of your chest, and out through your sitting bones. If properly balanced, you can raise either leg slightly without being forced to shift position noticeably.

This concept of sitting is a must to those of you who spend much time at a desk, if you wish to overcome headaches. It influences not only your basic stationary position, but the way you reach over the desk for telephone, books, notes, etc. Your body must pivot from the pelvic position, bending at the hips, not hunching over with shoulders and head thrust forward. When you reach forward, start pivoting right at your sitting bones, so that your lower back falls away from the back of your chair as your upper back does. On the other hand, this should *not* be interpreted as an absolutely rigid back, or the old "yardstick-down-the-back" concept taught years ago. The entire back should be flexible and mobile, but with most of the motion at the base of the spine, the upper back essentially retaining only its very modest curves.

Although posture is almost certainly a contributing factor in your headaches, *you cannot correct posture overnight.* Most headache victims are hard-working, well-motivated, self-disciplined individuals, and their first reaction to the above is to rush to work the next day convinced that they will keep themselves properly aligned all day, and by noon they are physical wrecks, stiff, tight, and sore. Please accept the fact that this is a slow conversion. If you have been sitting wrong for years, you cannot change it immediately, nor, more importantly, would you want to change it totally and immediately.

Why is this? The body has numerous position sensors and feedback circuits, and your body's sensors are tuned to your old ways. We want to achieve your posture correction not by having you tell yourself every ten seconds to "straighten up," but by having your sensors and feedback circuits gradually become attuned to your new positions so that control is firmly established subconsciously. Set up some sort of sequence consistent with your work patterns so that about once every hour you are reminded to check your body alignment.

While talking about sitting problems, we should not forget that old nemesis: the shoulders, probably an element in 60 to 80 percent of headaches. Again, we seek a neutral position. The key crimes: (1) shoulders rounded too far forward, stretching the back muscles and leading to "dowager's hump" because it is invariably accompanied by the head-forward position; (2) shoulders too far back, leading to the "pigeon breast" look and terrific tension between the shoulder blades; and (3) shoulders too high, the most serious and painful of all, because it constricts the trapezius muscle, which runs up the back of the neck, is tied directly to the back of the skull, and is implicated in virtually 100 percent of tension headaches.

Perhaps the most helpful concept is to realize that for both the chest and shoulders, good posture means "leave 'em alone!" The rib cage is, of course, hung from the spine, and is marvelously interconnected with small muscles so that the whole chest can swell and shrink. But precisely because of these interconnections, if the upper spine is properly erect, the chest will naturally assume its correct position, open and somewhat uplifted, not thrust out like a rooster, but neither so collapsed that the breastbone dives into the belly button.

There is one large exception to the "leave 'em alone" theory as it applies to the chest, and that is the postural problem of the concave chest. In this condition, the curvature of the upper back area is so pronounced and so ingrained that simply thinking the spine upright and straight, even coupled with the floor and wall straighteners, does not reprogram the body's reflex sensors. They are simply so conditioned to the old sensations that anything approaching correct spinal and chest alignment feels very strange, even painful. There are two approaches to this problem.

The Third Eye: The "third eye" concept is one that has been used successfully with some very recalcitrant postural problems. It is a game in which the player assumes that he or she has a third eye located in the breastbone, about a hand's width below the base of the neck. The game is that the third eye must be looking actively ahead of you at all times, standing or sitting. As you walk down the street, your third eye must be up and forward, scanning the path ahead; it plainly cannot do this if it is buried down inside your chest, looking at the ground! Perhaps this sounds silly as you read it, but give it an actual try. Play the role for even a few minutes and notice that as you move about, the concept may clash with some of your old established habits. If it does seem to make a difference, that certainly suggests that your regular alignment could stand some improvement.

The Lifted Rib Cage: A more direct approach is to be consciously aware of the rib cage, its elevation, and especially its distance above the waist. Women seem better at this direct approach than men, perhaps because their mode of dress makes them more aware of exactly where the waistline is. If the rib cage is kept clearly separated, "up and out of" the waist, then it will naturally be lifted and the upper spine straightened. The hazard that many males seem to be prone to with this approach is that they try to achieve chest lift by punching in the upper back, the exaggerated "military" look.

Now, using the chest as a clue, consider the shoulders once more, those beautifully engineered attachments. Remember that they are firmly attached to your torso at only one point: in the front, directly at the base of the neck, where your collarbones rest on your chest. To students of body language, the shoulders speak reams, just because of their great mobility. We can all conjure up images of friends and acquaintances whose shoulder positions immediately say: anger / fright /

nervousness / aggression / tension / fear / confidence / pride / etc. Of course, natural contours differ considerably, from very square to very sloping, and your natural position has to be based on your natural structure. The almost universal flaw is lifting the shoulders too much, putting stress on the neck and lower skull. If you need a position concept, think "wide." Get this feel by extending the arms to the side at shoulder level, then pressing the fingertips out as far as possible. Sense that, then lower the arms and use the same sense to imagine your shoulders extending out to the side, but do not raise them. Also, shrug your shoulders vigorously up and down and around, then let them settle down into a natural relaxed position.

I cannot exaggerate how important the habits of proper sitting and loose shoulders are to your headache problem. Just remember that you have this incredible computer and feedback system in your body that *will* remake your habits, *if* you will frequently give it the right encouragement.

THINK UPRIGHT
THINK TALL
THINK LOOSE

And now to walking, where the same elements are at work, with the same need for positive reinforcement. Again, the tilt of the pelvis is the vital key. The eternal problem is that the top of the pelvis slips forward, making the small of the back sink in and the derriere push back, causing the common "swayback." This also causes the abdomen to bulge forward, with the chest sinking on top of it. Pretty picture? Of course not, but sit down anytime and "people-watch" for a while and you will see the above description over and over. It's also called "Oh, my achin' back!"

So "tuck in your tail." If you have trouble with the concept, think of the way you would tuck in if you were squeezing sideways through a narrow opening. Another way to get the feeling very clearly is to locate a steep hill to walk down, even if only a short driveway or ramp. The natural adjustment your body will make to walking down is to tilt your pelvis under, lift the knee, and swing your leg from the hip, just exactly the effect you are looking for.

Now, with the pelvis properly adjusted, just assume the

plumb-line position: head-shoulders-chest-torso-pelvis, all lined up. But again, don't force it. Think it, relax, and walk. Then, in a little while, think it again.

If you are able to rig a traction collar, as described in chapter 8, the feeling while stretching can be easily and directly carried over to the walking and sitting posture concepts, because, when stretched, everything is lined up correctly.

Above all, keep mobile, all over. Good posture must not be confused with stiffness. You must always keep the feeling of good fluid motion, not only in gliding across the sidewalk, but in the various parts of your body. Walking is absolutely one of the finest all-around exercises you can do, so make the most of it. Swing your arms, letting your shoulders flow back and forth to counterbalance your stride. Keep your knees and ankles flexible. Lead with the knee-lift, pivoting at the hip joint, with the pelvis rotating slightly about the spine, so that as your left leg starts forward, the left side of the pelvis comes forward somewhat also. Then as the right leg takes over, the pelvis rotates, thrusting the right side forward. As with all things in posture, this must not be exaggerated—just a slight motion forward and back; it does wonders for fatigue if you really have a long way to walk.

Then, to that last problem area: standing. Nothing is more tiring for most of us than having to be on our feet, but not being free to really walk off and enjoy that motion we were just discussing. We stand until we slump, as if we were collapsing in a chair: pelvis tipped, stomach out, chest collapsed, shoulders rounded, head forward, neck muscles tightening, headache coming.

No, it doesn't need to come! Keep loose, keep moving. There is almost never a standing situation where we really have to remain absolutely motionless. Even a soldier at parade attention can achieve small muscle and joint movements without his uniform ever showing a thing. And in the average standing situation, behind a counter, waiting in a line, etc., we really are free to get all sorts of motion into our bodies on a small but very significant scale. If you feel yourself tiring or tensing, start with your feet and work up. Wiggle your toes, then rock slightly forward and back or side to side. Press your weight on the ball of one foot and then the other, then on the heels. Bend the knees slightly, together and then alternately; do the same at the hips. Contract the buttocks, then flex the all-important pelvis and rotate slightly. Bend slightly at the waist and take a deep breath to raise and lower the rib cage. Move the shoulders (a vital area) all around, forward-back, up-down, tense and relax; now the neck and head, forward-back (remember how a chicken walks?), rotate, tilt, *move!*

Then, when you really get a chance for a break, make the most of it. Don't flop in a chair and collapse. Move first. Two fine movements can be done in seconds. Spread feet, bend knees, put hands on knees with arms straight, lower torso until arms push shoulders up toward ears, then swing hips from side to side by bending in the waist so that the entire back and shoulders are stretched. Next stand tall, then lean forward from the waist, allowing the knees to bend comfortably as the head hangs forward. Hang arms down in front and shake them out. Only seconds to do, but what relief!

One final very important fact to bear in mind is that the "chest-up" posture has a *real* effect on your emotional state and your image of yourself. We are all familiar with the collapsed posture of depression; so much so that a cartoonist can convey the "people are no damned good" feelings of his character by changing only a few basic lines from the "walking on top of the world" figure. What we don't stop to realize is that assuming the posture of a confident buoyant personality in itself has a dramatic effect on our emotional state. Our emotions are fed continually by those same sensors that read our body position every second, and that input has a strong influence on our self-image.

This is a very basic animal trait, common to all higher animals, and one that owners of dogs will be particularly aware of, since dogs interact with one another very much by body language. Look at dogs on a street or playground and observe the changes of tail position, head and ears position, and occasionally the whole body shape, as small and large dogs interact. This is also strongly dependent on which dog is on his home territory, and who is the trespasser.

If you want to be confident, start by looking confident. You have a great body—even the worst body in the world is an absolutely magnificent machine, computer, and chemical factory—be proud of it.

The Alexander Method

One of the earliest modern contributions to what is now called "holistic" or "integral" medicine was that of F. M. Alexander. A brief review of his story offers an interesting and positive commentary on the role of "self-help" in medical problems. He was born in Tasmania, in 1869, and turned to a performing career as a "reciter of dramatic and humorous pieces." However, he began to develop serious problems with his voice, and very nearly lost his voice completely.

His consultations with physicians were not helpful, so he tackled the problem himself by carefully observing himself in front of a mirror while doing recitations. He became aware that his vocal problems worsened as he took stances which he had felt quite appropriate for the material he was reciting. Over a number of years he worked on what would probably now be called "body language," relating the various stances and movements to his vocal problem, eventually recovering completely.

With the awareness generated by the study of his own postures and movements, Alexander observed others, coming to realize that, indeed, most people stand, sit, and move in an equally defective manner. He began teaching actors how to use his remarkable discoveries—new concepts of how to move and position one's body. Then his teachings began to spread to a variety of people, and he finally trained a number of his pupils as teachers of his method.

The nonverbal teaching method uses the teacher's hands to gently position and move individual parts of the student's body. The student lies on his back on an unpadded table; the teacher starts with the head and neck, gradually working down the shoulders, back, chest, pelvis, legs, and feet. After a few sessions, some upright positions and movements are also introduced, gradually blended with the table work. This is done almost solely with the guidance of the teacher's hands.

Because the process is nonverbal, it would be most difficult to describe here, but several important points about it are well worth making. The first is that it is further confirmation of the vital fact that your body is *one* unit; all parts interact with all other parts, and to achieve really good health, *all parts must be tuned together.* Second, the end objective of the Alexander Method is to achieve good posture, and that improved posture is the key element in the therapeutic effects of the method. However, it must be emphasized again that good posture does not mean the military look that so many of us in this country associate with the term. It is as bad for the spine to be over-arched as for it to be slumped. The overall objective is a general straightness of the spine, except for the slight natural curves above the pelvis and in the chest area.

And last, one visualization that Alexander teachers use for body movement can be very helpful. It is to see yourself standing, sitting, and moving as if your head were suspended from a point directly above you, rather than feeling as if your head were simply plotched on top of your spine. We move and sit as if the head weighed 100 pounds and were pressing down on our entire body, bending the spine, compressing the chest, requiring us to push with our arms to even rise from a chair.

How different it would feel if there were an invisible wire attached to the topmost point of the skull, suspended from a freely moveable support directly over the head that carried all the weight of the head and even a little extra. In that case, the head would seem to actually have a buoyancy to it, like a helium-filled balloon, floating along above our shoulders. It would lift the entire body, pulling the neck up out of the shoulders, stretching and straightening the spine, lifting the rib cage, stretching the waist, and allowing the legs to flow beneath the body because the feet would feel so little pressure. Sounds marvelous, doesn't it?

Think lightness in the head; let your *head* lead you up out of the chair; let your *head* lift you along the sidewalk as you stride along. *Remember: it is literally all in the way you see yourself.*

Mechanics of Breathing

We all know how to breathe. Don't we? We need oxygen to live, so if we're alive we must be breathing, right? Perhaps. That's a little like saying that a car doesn't need a new air filter simply because it is running, even though the air filter may be visibly coated with dirt. Sure, it's getting air, but how efficiently?

You realize, of course, that we breathe by alternately increasing and decreasing the pressure inside of our lungs. After we decrease the pressure, outside air rushes in (inhalation). After we increase the pressure, some of the inside gas mixture, no longer air in terms of composition, flows out (exhalation).

The question is, how do we achieve that pressure change; with what muscles, and in what part of the lungs? The chest is beautifully constructed. It is a bellows; it is a piston and cylinder; and it is a combination of those devices.

The chest cavity is rather like a pyramid, or an inverted cone, with most of its volume at the bottom. The cone of the chest cavity is formed by the ribs, with the diaphragm forming the floor. That's where we should breathe from—the bottom. It's the natural place to breathe; watch any baby breathe and notice the abdominal movement. To inhale, we need to lower the pressure inside, and we can do that in two ways: lift and expand the walls of the cone (the chest), or lower the floor (the diaphragm). Most of us usually do the former, breathing shallowly and inefficiently, using the less effective upper part of the lungs. (The upper part of the lungs contains relatively more of the "pipes," the trachea and bronchial tubes, and less of the actual gas exchange vessels or alveoli.)

It is far healthier to breathe with the diaphragm and lower rib cage, so that the full lung is involved and active in oxygen exchange. This motion can be felt easily by placing one hand on the front of your stomach, just below the breastbone, and the other on your side, just above your waist. When you inhale naturally, the front of your stomach comes forward and the waist expands laterally. One of the worst consequences of poor posture is that with the body slumped forward it is almost impossible for the diaphragm and lower rib cage to do their job. If your posture is good, it is very easy to breathe naturally; conversely, if you are breathing naturally, your posture will tend to be better automatically.

How is all this related to headaches? Primarily because of the interaction with posture, and secondarily because of the more complete use of torso muscles involved in natural breathing. It all goes back to the concept that I keep hammering away at—"muscles are made for moving." Upper-chest breathing tends to result in raised, often locked, shoulders, and the resultant tensions inevitably drift up the neck to the head. In diaphragmatic breathing, the whole torso swells and shrinks, the shoulders gently lifting slightly, all the upper torso muscles smoothly and consistently interacting with one another, *without tension.* (Just stop to realize that breathing rate is a key index in lie detector tests.) *Breathing without tension is life without tension.*

Whole Body Conditioning

This is a key chapter for many headache victims. Read it carefully, and think even more carefully about how it relates to your way of life. There are three basic classes of benefits from exercise: physical, chemical, and emotional. I will discuss these separately, although they interact strongly with one another.

Physical: The effects most easily observed under this category are increases in strength and flexibility. The degree to which these appear is closely tied to the type of exercise performed, and, of course, any form of sports is included here. Tests have shown that some sports, such as bowling or golf (if carts are used), do very little for muscular strength. Sports like jogging, so very good in many ways, may decrease flexibility because of the limited motion involved. However, extremes of strength or flexibility have very little to do with the general health of your body. As you grow older, it is very important to try to minimize the loss of both flexibility and strength that gradually occurs with aging. Flexibility is probably the more important to retain because of its relation to relaxation of muscles, a key element in headache prevention.

The most important unseen physical effect of exercise is the multifaceted benefit to circulation. For example, vigorous exercise leads to increased vascularity; that is, the body will actually develop additional capillaries (the ultrafine blood vessels that connect the arteries to the veins) in muscle and other tissues as a response to the activity. This permits better delivery of oxygen to the tissues and more prompt removal of waste products from the tissues, an important factor in preventing muscle stiffness.

Physical activity has a very strong "heart-sparing" effect. In fact the large thigh muscles have been described as a "second heart" because of their role in pumping blood back to the heart whenever they are alternately contracted and relaxed, as in any type of walking or running. This minimizes pooling of blood in the legs and in the inner organs, and the ill effects that pooling can produce.

Last, the benefits of full body exercise are felt in the lungs and chest, particularly if the effort is strenuous enough to require really deep breathing. If not, as in slower walking, then deep breathing can be practiced voluntarily during the walk to produce most of the same benefits. These include increased circulation through the lungs; the massaging motion of the diaphragm and abdominal muscles on the inner organs; and full opening of the rib cage. The latter is very important to, improved posture and headache prevention. As one grows older, the rib cage begins to lose its flexibility, and often starts to lock into a position that holds the chest down and the head forward. Regular deep breathing will do much to alleviate this condition.

Chemical: This is a complicated subject, but you need only appreciate that the metabolic chemical by-products of exercise are really constructive agents to your well-being. Their effects range from improving the efficiency of your body to improving your mood. Many of the effects of physical training, such as the increase in your stamina, are derived from increases in the efficiency with which the blood absorbs, carries, and releases oxygen to the tissues. Efficiency also improves for the process of removing the waste products and transporting them to the lungs, liver, and kidneys, where their metabolism is completed.

Your body is really a very finely tuned system, with many interlocking feedback mechanisms, in which biochemical molecules act as the messengers to indicate changes, needs, excesses, etc. Regular "revving up" of your system, as happens in good physical activity, has a tremendous normalizing effect on all of your subsystems and produces the proper levels and distributions for all of these chemical messengers.

Emotional: Perhaps the most important benefits to headache victims fall into this category, because headaches are closely related to our emotional state. The effects here arise from both of the above categories, i.e., physical and chemical. Feedback from our muscles, the so-called kinesthetic sense, can have a direct effect on how we feel about ourselves. How we view our bodies is often the way we feel others see us; a change in posture and/or muscle tone can have a striking effect on how we see the world and how the world sees us.

The chemical changes can also have a direct and immediate effect on our mood. You should be aware that your own body produces true "mood-altering" chemicals, just like the ones that have received so much publicity in recent years. If you can eliminate your depression by a quick game of tennis or a brisk walk, that is not all in your mind, in the sense that it just makes you forget your troubles. One way of looking at it is that it produces actual chemical changes in your brain, which you then perceive as changes in your mood or in the nature of your troubles.

An important factor to bear in mind is that the exercise you choose should be something you truly enjoy. And I mean *truly* enjoy, all the way through. There is no point to looking forward to walking around the golf course, or to hitting a tennis ball with a friend, if you are going to become so upset at losing or at bad shots that you finish the game more frustrated or angry than when you began. And if you choose a nongame, such as jogging or swimming, you may have the same trouble if you are doing it *only* because you know it is "good" for you! Forcing yourself may do more harm than good.

At this point, please review in your mind your physical activities in recent months. Be honest with yourself about how you feel after most of your games or outings. Are you uptight because you lost, or didn't play well, or just plain didn't enjoy it? If so, you should consider another form of activity for a while. Keep looking; there are a multitude of physical activities, and you are bound to find one that you truly enjoy.

This enjoyment can take many forms or can occur at different phases. Thus, it may arise less from your love of the game than from your pleasure in the company the game produces. Or perhaps you find it a grind in itself, but love the afterglow feeling. The variety of exercise is endless, but it should be something you can do several times a week that leads to an increased pulse rate and some increase in breathing rate and volume. Very strenuous exercise once a week is not nearly as good as even less exertion three times a week.

Exercise should definitely involve your legs. I will not try to itemize all forms, but swimming, jogging, and serious biking are extremely good. The one simple exercise available to us all, and which has proven to be of immense benefit, is walking. It is also a form which can be included in your daily routine with little loss of time, if you will give the matter some thought. The automobile has probably done more damage to American health than any other hazard, because it has eliminated so much short-distance walking. But with a little thought, you can add just that kind of walking back into your life. Don't rush out and sell your car—simply stop using it for every short trip you make. And if you must use it, for shopping, for example, park out at the end of the parking lot opposite the store you plan to visit, and *walk*. If you travel by bus, get off somewhat before or after your regular stop, and make up the difference on foot.

Several very fine books on exercise are listed in the bibliography (including a really superb one on walking). *Walk* down to your local library and browse through some of them.

CHAPTER 7

Relax!

Alpha Rhythms

It has been known for many years that a specific state of relaxation of the body muscles results in a frequency of electrical activity in the brain known as alpha waves, or alpha rhythms. It was then proposed that this relationship could be reversed: if one could induce the brain to produce alpha waves, the body musculature would relax.

Experiments have shown that this is basically true, although it may not be cause and effect; that is, it may simply be that the same conditions that lead to an alpha state also lead to muscular relaxation. But, from a practical standpoint, that question is irrelevant. If we wish to achieve a certain end result, it is not necessary to fully understand just why it works, just that it does work.

There are various methods of achieving the alpha state, most of them unnecessarily complicated. Perhaps the most common, in terms of numbers of students, is transcendental meditation (TM), which uses as its core a "mantra," which is a word or sound that has no meaning in the English language. In a twenty-minute meditation, this mantra may be repeated a thousand times or more, a situation cheerfully accepted by some, but which others find highly aggravating.

There is, fortunately, a much simpler method of achieving

the same or, in fact, better results with a technique you can learn in ten minutes or so. All methods are based on a common fact. You do not "put yourself into alpha"; instead you simply "allow your brain to shift itself into alpha." All methods have in common that you are directed to concentrate on something; in TM it's the mantra, in others a familiar place or object, until the brain "changes gears."

In our method, you visualize a very simple series of numbers. Why numbers? Because we see them every day, on TV, in the papers, on license plates, etc. The simple sequence? Well, it's 3—2—1; nothing could be much simpler than that. The process is as follows:

(Read the full chapter before trying the process.)

First: Sit erect in a comfortable chair, feet on floor, hands in lap, but separated (not folded together).

Second: Close eyes and visualize an outside location you know very well, such as your backyard, the street in front of your home, an empty golf course or tennis court with which you are very familiar; in other words, a scene you can clearly visualize.

Third: Breathing normally, but remaining conscious of your breathing rate, visualize the following numbers in sequence on the location you are visualizing, seeing the numbers change progressively with *each* breath. The numbers are: a large 3, a medium 3, a small 3; a large 2, a medium 2, a small 2; a large 1, a medium 1, a small 1.

Example: I visualize the front street of a home where we lived for many years. Across the street are some tall palm trees, in front is a mailbox on a post. These serve as references as follows: For each large number, such as the large 3, I visualize a 3 as tall as the palm trees, curving from the tops right down to the ground. For the medium 3, I see a 3 the height of the mailbox (obviously much smaller than the first 3). For the small 3, I see the 3 on the license plate of my car sitting in the driveway (again, a significant decrease in size). Then I see the 2s in the same places in sequence, remembering to change numbers only with each exhalation, breathing normally but rather slowly. I continue with the three sizes of 1s and when I finish the small 1, I say to myself silently (just in my mind): "Now I am in a shallow alpha. I am very relaxed, and my head is cool and calm. My hands and arms are heavy, I can feel gravity pulling them down against my lap, making them relax. My head . . . neck . . . and shoulders are cool and relaxed . . . very cool and very relaxed. Now I am going deeper into alpha."

At this point, you will indeed be in a light alpha. To go into a deeper alpha, you proceed as follows: Take a moderately deep breath (this is one reason you want to be sure to sit erectly in the beginning) and hold it. Then slowly and silently count from ten down to one; with each count down you will go deeper into the alpha state. After one, exhale slowly, breathe naturally, and take advantage of your alpha state. How? By using autosuggestions, i.e., implanting constructive statements that will continue to work through your subconscious mind after you rouse yourself. Caution: you must use only *positive* statements, no negative statements. For example, instead of "my head does not hurt," say "my head feels fine."

Just the act of going into the alpha state twice a day will do great things for your well-being, self-confidence, and self-image, in addition to your tension and headache relief. However, alpha can be used most effectively if you use a sequence of self-implanted suggestions that relate to your particular needs, desires, problems, etc. For example, if tension headaches are your problem (aren't they everybody's?) you might use statements like:

"I am very calm and relaxed."

"I really enjoy my work and look forward to it."

"I really look forward to the kids coming home from school."

"My head feels loose and relaxed; my forehead is loose and relaxed; my neck is loose and relaxed."

Obviously the autosuggestion technique can be used for many things, including other physical ailments and/or emotional problems, but our objective now is to eliminate your headaches, so here is a sequence of statements to be used in the final stages of your alpha period:

"My forehead is relaxed."

"My temples are relaxed."

"The scalp above my ears is relaxed."

"The scalp at the back of my head is relaxed."

"The upper part of my neck is relaxed."

"The lower part of my neck is relaxed."

"My shoulders are relaxed."

You may well choose different words to select the parts of your head and neck. The only important thing is to use a regular progression from one part to the next adjacent part. Use words you are comfortable with and understand (anatomical names might be meaningless to some). Say them to yourself, silently, at a slow and measured pace, thinking about each part of the head and neck as you are describing its relaxed condition.

Instead of the word "relaxed," you may wish to use something else, such as "loose," or "cool," whatever is most comfortable. You do not need to use exactly the same words or sequence each time, although some people find it better if their procedure is very structured.

To close the alpha period, we use a "count-up" sequence. You say to yourself (always silently, of course):

"Now I am going to come out of the alpha state; I will count up from one to five, and when I reach five I will be wide awake. I will be calm, rested, relaxed, and feeling very good. One . . Two . . . . . Three . . . . Four . . . . Five." As the dots suggest, the count-up should be slow, with a slight increase in pause between each number. After five, and before opening your eyes, stretch by extending your arms and opening and closing your hands several times.

Although this procedure is lengthy to describe, performing an alpha need take only a few minutes, although to be most effective, one should spend about five minutes. If you have difficulty visualizing, as some people do, find some large numbers in print, e.g., magazine or newspaper ads, and for the first few sessions look at these numbers directly before closing the eyes for a session.

Very Important: Do *not* expect to feel some strange or peculiar sensation in the alpha state. It is a perfectly normal state, which you pass through several times during a normal night's sleep. You might be aware of it only as that particularly pleasant period when you are half-awake when sleeping late on a Saturday morning, or in just drifting off to sleep at night.

One caution, which may sound strange at first: be sure to visualize your space, where you will see the numbers, free of any moving objects, such as cars, people, dogs, etc. Remember that when you visualize, your imagination is not totally restrained, only focused, and this may influence your choice of a location. For example, someone who lives on a busy street, and who chooses the front yard with perhaps the telephone pole across the street to project his "big 3" may suddenly find cars whizzing by in front of the telephone pole! Obviously that will be very distracting and will interfere with the alpha, so pick a location that you feel comfortable seeing completely empty of moving objects.

Also, pick an image where you can "see" all of the numbers without having to move your point of view. One learner tried to use her front yard, including her house number for the small numbers, but because she was "standing on the porch" (her point of view), she had to "turn around" to see the small number of each sequence. This badly interrupts the process. Pick a location and point of view where you can easily see each number of the sequence as they blend from one to the next.

Please try this method. It can be *very* important to your headaches. Take advantage of that fantastic computer you have between your ears. If you reprogram it properly, it will do absolute wonders for you.

Relaxation

Relaxation is a vital factor in most headaches. Perhaps that should read "lack of relaxation" is a vital factor in most headaches. Tension is a contributing factor in almost every headache, so relaxation methods that effectively reduce tension are important in headache control. Relaxation, as it is used here, refers to both muscular and emotional tensions, since they cannot be fully separated in the human body. One simply *cannot* get tense emotionally without producing muscle tension, and vice versa.

Our methods of brushing, alpha, massage, and posture control will definitely reduce both types of tension, but we will discuss here some additional well-tested methods for producing relaxation, which, at your option, can be included in your program. I will give you specific directions for using the Jacobson Progressive Relaxation Method, Autogenic Feedback Training, Chromatherapy, and discuss some of the pros and cons of biofeedback.

The Jacobson Method: Dr. E. Jacobson published this technique in the late 1930s, and it has been used with great success in many applications since then. It is based on the concept that although we may find it difficult to specifically *relax* a muscle, we all have the ability to *tense* a particular muscle group. The method works as follows:

Lie on your back on a firm surface, either a very firm bed or the floor, with a pillow under your head and another under your knees, so that the legs are slightly bent. Adjust both pillows so that you are very comfortable. Now focus your attention on your right foot. Tense all the muscles in your right foot until they are really firm and pulling against one another, then suddenly relax them completely. Now address your right calf and lower leg, and repeat the same sequence: tighten, and then suddenly relax. Next the right thigh. You should be able to get a good strong tightening here, probably with much more feeling than in the lower leg. Hold for a second, then let the muscles collapse. At this point, the whole right leg should feel really limp, just totally relaxed.

Now turn to the left foot with the same procedure, then the left calf, and the left thigh. Next the right buttock, and then the left. Then the abdominals, the lower back, and the upper back. Here do the right side first, including the chest muscles and back muscles together, then go to the left side. Now start with the right hand, then the forearm, the upper arm, and the shoulder. Now move to the left hand, and follow the same sequence up through the left shoulder. I find the trapezius and neck best done as a unit at this point, but be sure you feel the tension all the way from the tops of the shoulders into the head, both front and back. Relax your body completely, and do your jaw muscles, face, and scalp. As you practice this sequence, you will find you can subdivide large muscle groups into smaller groups that you can contract and relax at will, thus giving you more and more control over your body. When you have completed the sequence, rest for about five minutes (totally relaxed), then have a really good, satisfying stretch, roll over, and slowly get to your feet.

In times of need, you will find that once you have practiced this method, you can use parts of it advantageously when sitting or standing. Thus, even if you are in a meeting and you feel tension coming on, you can, quietly and with no visible motion, tighten selected muscle groups individually, drop them into a relaxed state, and lower your whole tension level. You will naturally think of doing your neck and shoulders because of the obvious relation to headaches, but do not forget the large thigh and buttock muscles, as these are very important to blood circulation, especially when sitting for long periods of time.

Autogenic Feedback Training: This derives from the work of Drs. J. H. Schultz and W. Luthe in the late 1960s. They described a series of psychophysiologically oriented approaches that, in contrast to other medical or psychological forms of treatment, involve the simultaneous regulation of mental and somatic (body) functions. In this technique, as modified at the Menninger Clinic by Dr. Joseph D. Sargent, the objective was to train the patient to achieve general relaxation of the body and an increased blood flow to the hands. The ability to "think" increased blood flow to the hands was shown to improve migraine headaches in a sizeable percentage of victims.

The method simply involves the repetition of phrases specifically designed to achieve the desired effects. The subject first memorizes the phrases. Then, while seated very comfortably with the eyes closed, the subject recites the phrases silently while visualizing the changes actually taking place in his body. The Menninger group was interested primarily in migraines, but the technique is applicable to other headaches also. Their sequence of phrases is as follows:

> *I feel quite quiet. . . . I am beginning to feel quite relaxed. . . . My feet feel heavy and relaxed. . . . My ankles, my knees, and my hips feel heavy, relaxed, and comfortable. . . . My solar plexus, and the whole central portion of my body, feel relaxed and quiet. . . . My hands, my arms, and my shoulders feel heavy, relaxed, and comfortable. . . . My neck, my jaws, and my forehead feel relaxed. . . . They feel comfortable and smooth. . . . My whole body feels quiet, heavy, comfortable, and relaxed. I am quite relaxed. . . . My*

arms and hands are heavy and warm. . . . I feel quite quiet. . . . My whole body is relaxed and my hands are warm, relaxed and warm. . . . My hands are warm. . . . Warmth is flowing into my hands, they are warm . . . warm.

Chromatherapy: The use of color in healing goes back to the Egyptians and Greeks. The Hindus also have used it for years, and there are color practitioners in many parts of Europe. My purpose in introducing it here is for general relaxation, and particularly for those of you who may have trouble visualizing specific shapes and details such as are used in some other methods. "Color breathing" is done by closing your eyes and imagining that you are engulfed in a colored cloud; as you breathe slowly, the color flows into your body and moves where you see it. Inhale slowly for four counts, retain the breath (and the color) for eight counts, and slowly exhale for four counts allowing the color to flow out. Do this four times. You should select a color comfortable to you, or let one come. If you are nervous, blue is a good choice. A natural outdoor green is always a calming color to use, and easily visualized. This is a method that can be readily used almost anywhere, and could be one of your "bag of tricks" for future needs.

Biofeedback: This is not a method for you to use by yourself since, if done properly, it involves some fairly sophisticated electronic equipment. However, a brief review of the subject will be helpful in your understanding of the concept of headache control. Biofeedback started with investigations of the EEG (electroencephalograph), or electrical waves produced by the brain as recorded from the scalp. There are basically four types of waves: alpha, beta, delta, and theta, each of a different frequency and voltage. It was thought for many years that these waves were purely a reflection of the state of the brain and nervous system (i.e., waking, sleeping, resting, etc.) and quite independent of the personal control of the individual. However, in the 1960s, workers such as Dr. Joseph Kamiya began to note that some individuals could exercise a degree of control over their brain waves. More important to us, it was shown that with practice, almost everyone could learn to control his EEG to some degree. Scientists then began to look at heart rate, and found that people could raise and lower that at will, with some training. Blood pressure could also be lowered, just by thinking about lowering it. At first this concept was not well received, as it flew in the face of classic medical science, but now it is an accepted fact, and biofeedback is used at many medical centers today. This is living proof that *your mind can control your body.*

CHAPTER 8

Getting the Kinks Out

Orthopedic Collars

There are two types of orthopedic collars that are important to consider using if your headaches are in the slightest way related either to poor postural alignment or to tension in the neck or shoulder muscles.

Cervical Collars: The first type to consider using is known as a "cervical collar" and comes in a wide variety of shapes and materials. They are sold by medical supply shops but may require a prescription in some states. I suggest first trying the larger discount drug chains, as many of them carry the simple models, which are most appropriate for this use. The most effective inexpensive type is a felt or foam strip about four inches wide inside a woven cotton stocking. The collar is wrapped around the neck to a comfortable shape and degree of tension, and fastened with either a safety pin or an attached Velcro® fastener.

This collar supplies immediate support to the head, removing stress from the neck muscles that hold the head in position. Relief is usually felt immediately, and this, of course, confirms the role of muscle stress in the headache process. This in turn implies a posture source, either from basic poor posture; a postural problem at work (e.g., leaning over a desk continually); or perhaps a muscular weakness from illness, injury, or abuse.

The collar should *not* be used for long periods too frequently, for it can easily become a crutch. Its purpose in our application is to afford *temporary* relief, and break up the vicious circle of posture-tension-headache. Initially it should be used for perhaps thirty minutes in the late morning and a similar time in the late afternoon. You will quickly learn to judge the effects and benefits yourself, but do not use it as a continuous crutch. You must develop proper neck strength and posture yourself and regard the collar as a "means to an end," not as "an end in itself." However, the value of these collars for many headache victims cannot be overstated. I personally carry mine in my suitcase whenever I travel, because after a long period in a car or airplane, where movement is limited, a brief period with the collar will do wonders to relieve the neck muscles and break up tension.

Traction Collars: The second type of orthopedic collar is the "traction collar" and, as the name suggests, it is used to apply traction to the whole head in order to effectively lengthen the neck, straighten the cervical (neck) vertebrae, and, in fact, straighten the whole spine. These collars can be purchased at any medical supply shop, usually located in the Yellow Pages under the heading "Hospital Equipment and Supplies."

First, you must supply an overhead mounting point, using a large hook obtainable at any hardware store or home improvement center. The hook should be of a type at least five inches long, and with a shaft diameter of 5/16". Mount this hook overhead, *making sure it is screwed into a ceiling joist,* not just into the plaster. A good location is often in the garage, since garage joists can be easily seen. You will also need a length of quarter-inch rope, preferably nylon or dacron. The rope needs to be four times as long as the distance from your neck to the hook when you stand directly under it.

To mount the traction collar, tie each end of the rope to one of the rings at the top of the traction collar; then loop the doubled-up rope over the hook. Now double the end loop of the rope on itself and insert a short wooden rod, such as a piece of broomstick. You now have the rope over the hook, with the traction collar hanging on one side and the handle hanging on the other.

Orthopedic collars

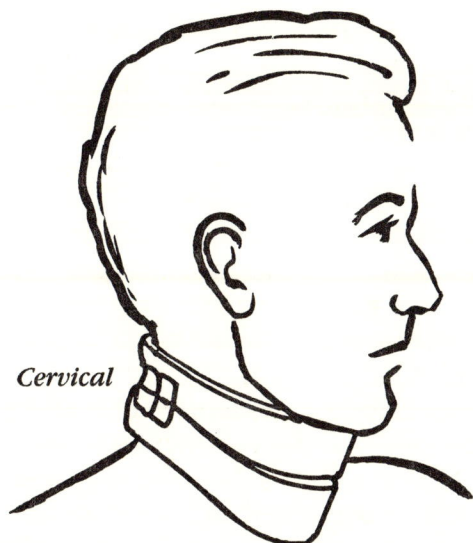

Cervical

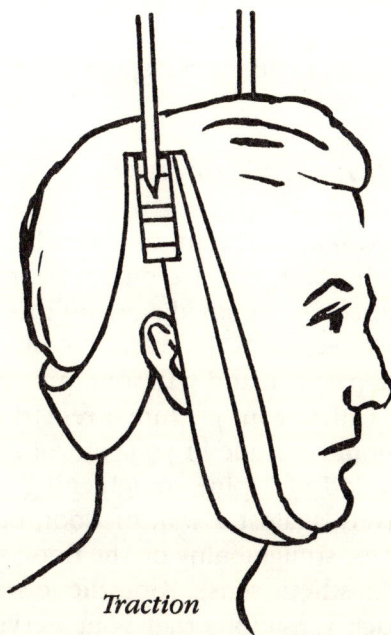

Traction

The traction collar is used as follows: Stand directly under the hook and connect the collar around the chin and neck. Pull down on the handle until the collar is firm and comfortable around the neck. (NOTE: to prevent any stress on the teeth, keep the pressure mainly on the back of the neck and the base of the jaw. Keep the mouth slightly open, so that the teeth are not quite in contact.) Now slowly pull down on the handle while slowly rising on the balls of your feet. When fully on the balls of your feet, keep a firm grip on the handle and gradually let your weight settle toward your heels by reducing the pressure on the balls of your feet. This, of course, puts tension on the head, lifting it from the torso in the exact direction desired. A light steady pull, continued for an initial ten seconds, and gradually working up to thirty seconds, will work wonders (exact times are not important; simply count to yourself). Repeat two or three times with a brief rest of half a minute or so between stretches. This process should be done twice a day, and is most effective if done shortly after arising in the morning, when the vertebrae are loose and adjustable, and again before dinner or at the end of the work day, when the vertebrae will be the most compressed and misaligned. Incidentally, in a few months, you will find that this procedure has added one-quarter to three-quarters of an inch to your height. This is proof indeed that stretching is effectively re-aligning your upper spine.

Spine Straightening

If you are reluctant to make the investment in a traction collar right away, or have difficulty arranging for the support hook, please start immediately on this alternative approach. It is not as effective as the traction collar, but it can be started with no preparation and will soon produce favorable results.

Unless your posture is remarkably good (a rarity today), you should include in your morning and evening program a short period of "spine straightening." This can be done very effectively against a wall or door, but should be preceded by the same straightening on the floor, so that you develop the proper kinesthetic sense. Kinesthetic sense refers to the postural feedback sensations that your nervous system receives from the position sensors distributed throughout your body. It is the development of this sense that leads to the unconscious stabilization of good posture.

Start by lying on your back on the floor, with the back of your head directly on the floor or carpet, knees bent so that the soles of your feet can comfortably rest flat on the floor. Now reach up over your head with your arms so that your elbows are close to your head and the backs of your hands are brushing the floor. You may have some difficulty at first in getting your arms straight *and* close to the floor. Do not force them. Simply come as close as is comfortable. Keeping the elbows straight, move your arms until they are extending laterally out from your shoulders. Be sure that the backs of the hands stay close to the floor or carpet during this swing. Slowly return to the original arm position and repeat three times. Now place the arms comfortably at your sides. Sense where your back, neck, and head are now. Feel under the small of your back with one hand and see how much space there is between your spine and the floor. Now remove your hand, and try to gently lower the small of your back to the floor. You will notice that it is much easier if you relax the neck and chest, letting them compensate naturally for the straightening of the spine. The chest will arch somewhat, the chin will sink in, and the head will probably tilt forward slightly, as if you were getting taller. Feel this position and the sensations it creates, and try to remember them. Do this several times, then relax for a moment. Get up slowly.

Now find the wall or door you plan to use, and back up to it. Move your feet out so that your heels are about twelve inches from the wall. Bring the back of your head to the wall while bending your knees slightly, and begin to press the small of your back toward the wall. Remember the sensations from your floor position. Do not force! We are simply stretching the vertebrae slightly, to get them separated as much as possible. *Think tall,* so that as your back comes in toward the wall, your head seems to grow toward the ceiling. With practice, you can start bringing your heels in closer to the wall, but always keep the knees bent slightly. Remember that in ideal posture, the spine has several natural curves, and we always want to stand and move with those curves in their natural place, not exaggerated. This spine straightening does tend to minimize the curvatures, and it provides the separation of the vertebrae that we are so anxious to achieve. It is a great break from either being on your feet too long or being cramped over your work too long. Take a few minutes each day and try it; exercises like this are their own reward.

Inverted Positions

In several places in this book, we stress the importance of the blood vessels of the head in relation to your headaches. The general circulation of the scalp, forehead, and neck is vital to your well-being. Many of our methods are aimed at improving the circulation, tone, and flexibility of the vessels. One very simple approach to that objective is through the use of inverted positions, in other words, upside down.

Gravity is usually an enemy of good circulation in your body. It drains the blood from your head, and pools it in your torso and legs. Inverted positions, on the other hand, allow you to put gravity to work in the right direction for a change, draining that pooled blood out of your extremities and increasing the flow to your entire head, especially the brain. The increased oxygen and the flushing out of metabolic waste from the brain are very refreshing and stimulating.

One very important caution: if you have any serious medical problems, such as high blood pressure, or have suffered a stroke in the past, do not use these positions without obtaining approval from your physician. If you are past forty, start these positions slowly, being particularly careful to rise slowly after the inverted position, lest some transient dizziness occur. The positions are listed in order of increasing difficulty.

Leg Elevation: This consists of placing your head and torso on a flat surface—the floor, a bed, or couch—then raising the legs up against the wall, the knees straight (or slightly bent, if more comfortable). You will thus be lying on your back, with your legs at nearly a right angle to your body. This is a very comfortable position, and you should be able to hold it for three to five minutes, more if you like.

Incline Board: If you have access to an incline board, such as is used for sit-up exercises, this is a great way to get a moderately inverted position that can be held for some time. It has an advantage over the first position: the head is lower than the torso, and the back is well supported.

Hang Off Bed: One way to get the head lower than the torso without equipment is to lie across the bed with your shoulders at the edge of the mattress and allow the head to fall back. You can do this first with your entire body and legs on the bed. Then, after a few times, raise the legs up onto the wall to increase the gravitational effect. An alternate position is to lie on your stomach with your head over the edge of the bed.

Shoulder Stand: This is a more advanced position, but possibly many of you are already doing it in exercise or yoga classes. There are several ways to get into this position, but here is one of the easiest. Sit on the floor with your knees well bent and your feet flat on the floor. Grasp under your thighs, just above the back of the knees. Round your back and roll backward, pulling your knees with you. As you roll toward your shoulders, straighten your knees somewhat and transfer your hands to your upper hips, with your elbows on the floor. Now extend your feet toward the ceiling, while working your elbows in closer to your body and pressing your hips upward. When balanced, this is a very comfortable position. It has the added advantage of flexing the back and neck nicely. Practice getting the body as elevated as possible, with just the neck flexed.

Head Stand (Yoga Version): Many of you may be familiar with this position. One kneels, bringing the top of the head to the floor. The hands are clasped, fingers interlocked, and placed around the back of the head, with the elbows and forearms on the floor. There are two schools of thought at this point; in both, the beginner practices in the corner of a room, against the intersection of two walls. The first school says to walk your feet toward your head until the buttocks are well elevated—the feet will naturally follow up and overhead. Depending on personal flexibility, some will find it easier to flip the fanny and legs up in one quick (but not violent!) motion. The best approach depends considerably on your personal build and condition.

Head Stand (Gym Version): Many of us were taught at some point in grade school to do this version, but may have forgotten it by now, so I'll give a quick review. Squat down with the feet about shoulder width apart. Place your hands on the floor, palms down, the same width apart as your feet, and with your elbows against your knees. Now rock forward, flexing the elbows but keeping them against your knees until your feet come off the ground and you are balanced on your hands. Let your head sink slowly to the floor, and swing the legs up overhead. Men are usually better at this type of head stand because of stronger arms, while women are often better at the yoga head stand because of better flexibility. Both are very good for you.

Caution: Keep in mind that if you have not used these positions in exercise programs recently, you should progress slowly. These are not to be madly rushed through, but to be savored and enjoyed. We headache people are often very impatient about "wasting time." *There is nothing wasteful about any time that is spent improving your health and well-being.* If you must, put on the radio. But most of all, relax and enjoy a few minutes of peace and quiet.

CHAPTER 9

Food, Temperature, and Light

Nutrition

Nutritional factors probably have a role in many headaches, although it is usually only a secondary role. Among migraine victims, it is common to have a sensitivity to one or more foods. These may include frankfurters (and other preserved foods containing nitrites), chocolate, peanuts, cocoa, rich cakes and cookies, cheeses like cheddar that contain tyramine, and fried foods. Tension headaches, which represent well over 80 percent of all headaches, are rarely precipitated directly by food substances.

However, a poor diet makes the body susceptible to all kinds of illness, and headaches are no exception. Headaches are primarily a reflection of stress. Stress is the sum total of all the insults to which our body is subjected daily; hence, each individual stress adds together to create the total stress. And the typical American diet is enough to stress anyone!

We eat *too much,* especially too much fats and sugar, and distribute the intake poorly throughout the day. Ideally, we should direct our diet to a moderately high protein level, a modest carbohydrate level, and a low fat level. The intake should be distributed fairly evenly over the day, with a good breakfast, satisfactory lunch, and a modest dinner, especially if the rest of the evening is to be spent in front of the television set. (The typical sequence is almost no breakfast, too much lunch, and much too much dinner!)

The bibliography includes several books relating to nutrition, and this is a subject on which everyone should become somewhat informed. Vitamin supplements are certainly appropriate for most of us, especially vitamins C and the B complex. Both have been shown to be constructive in headache syndromes. Vitamin C is related to blood circulation, among other things. The B complex is essential to intermediary metabolism, the digestion and transformation of food at a molecular level.

The book by Dr. Roger Williams is one you certainly should read, as he shows clearly how individualistic our needs are for specific vitamins. In a chemical sense, *you are not identical to any other individual on the face of this earth*—you are truly unique. Think about that, and you will realize that no one else can tell you exactly what you should eat. You must bear the responsibility of watching your intake of foods and carefully observing your reactions, especially as it relates to your headaches. *You are, after all, your own ultimate physician.*

Niacin

We have talked at considerable length about the relationship between headaches and peripheral circulation, a vital relationship both to your understanding and to your prevention of headaches. The arteries and arterioles, even the capillaries of your scalp and forehead, are the main causes of your headaches, but also offer you a surefire pathway to cure them. Anything that improves and normalizes the blood flow in your head will favorably affect your headache syndrome.

Niacin will definitely affect the circulation in your head. It is one of the water-soluble vitamins of the B complex, and was first made famous as a cure for the notorious ailment known as pellagra, especially prevalent in the southern states years ago. It is involved in cellular metabolism and is a part of all living cells, so a well-balanced diet should readily supply sufficient amounts of niacin.

However, in this day of processed and snack foods, it is no longer easy to obtain a really well balanced diet. Therefore, I definitely advise vitamin supplements, a general complete multivitamin being taken every day, preferably with breakfast.

If, at the same time, one takes 50 mg. of niacin, within the next thirty minutes a general flushing and heating of the face and scalp, as well as the rest of the body, will be felt as the capillaries dilate and blood accelerates through them. You will observe this effect only if you use niacin; the niacinamide form, though equally effective as a vitamin, produces no flushing whatsoever. The immediate effect is transient, with the skin returning to its normal color tones within another five minutes or so. The flush will vary somewhat in intensity from day to day, but will often be quite obvious, so time your intake so that family members or coworkers are not alarmed by your sudden blush!

Heat and Cold

Thermal methods can be very constructive both before and during a headache. Generally speaking, it is *heat* during the early first symptom stages and *cold* during the peak of the headache. But remember, there are strong individual differences in response, and you must monitor your own reaction to heat and cold. One way to remember the sequence is that it is the reverse of the approved treatment for a sprain or muscle pull. With a sprain, you apply cold immediately to minimize swelling, then start heat applications the next day to increase circulation and speed healing.

Heat: Warmth can be applied by an electric heating pad, hot water bottle, or towel or washcloth wrung out with hot water. If you use an electric pad, you may do better with some of the small, flexible ones that can be applied closely to the back of the neck or forehead. A hot water bottle conforms nicely to the shape of your head, but be careful to position it and yourself so that no extra weight is being supported by your neck. A wet towel or washcloth has the advantage that moist heat seems to penetrate the body better. If you are treating the back of the neck and upper shoulders, a soak in a hot tub can be very relaxing, providing you support your head properly against a small pillow or folded towel so that you can really completely relax the neck muscles.

One excellent way of routinely loosening up the neck and shoulder muscles with heat is to modify your shower

procedure slightly. Adjust the water temperature to as hot as
you can stand; then back under the water so that it plays directly on the back of your neck. Now rock from side to side so
that the water impinges on the trapezius on both sides. A short
session of this will do wonders for congestion in the neck and
shoulder area.

Heat has two basic effects. It increases blood flow by dilating the capillaries and simultaneously relaxes the muscles.
Since most headaches start with a reduction of blood flow, this
is a direct countermeasure to the initial problem. Application
of heat to the back of the neck and the temples will often improve conditions sufficiently to arrest the development of the
headache. One unlikely point to consider for heat is the exact
top of the head. It is not connected to the muscular areas, but
can sometimes produce great relief, because one of the main
headache acupressure points is located there. Of course, if
there is any reason to suspect sinus involvement, heat should
be applied to the areas above and below the eyes. Lie on your
side, with the most congested sinus on the upper side, so that
drainage can occur.

Cold: This treatment can best be done with a gel-type cold
pack, available at most drugstores. They can be kept indefi-
nitely in a freezer compartment for ready availability, are soft
so they conform to the body shape, and hold their chill for a
long treatment. Dr. Leo Diamond, the dean of American headache clinicians, has recently reported good results in migraine
relief with cold treatment.

If a gel pack is not available, a plastic bag will serve very ade-
quately. Put in some crushed ice cubes and about a half-cup of
water. The water is very important as it provides for good thermal contact with the surface of the body. Twist the top of the
bag, fold it over, and secure with a rubber band. Because the
plastic is so thin, you will need a washcloth between the bag
and your skin for comfort. If the washcloth seems to keep you
from feeling the cold, wet it first and it will make a better thermal transfer.

Cold has two effects. It reduces the circulation by decreasing the size of the capillaries and arteries, and reduces the sensitivity of the pain nerve endings. All biological processes slow
as the temperature drops, so the irritation of metabolic chemical products is also reduced. The cold can be applied to the

spots where you feel the pain, or to points such as the back of the neck or top of the head.

Please bear in mind that in addition to using heat and cold for immediate problems, they can be of great value in preventing a critical situation from arising. Since the muscles of the back of the neck and head are involved in so many headaches, the regular application of heat, at an appropriate time during the day, will often prevent a critical situation from ever arising. Consider your work or home situation, and see if there may be a period when you are particularly inclined to tenseness, and when a five-minute application of heat would break up the inevitable vicious circle.

Bright Light

Many headache victims mention their sensitivity to light, both before and during an attack. Ordinary room lights can seem like intense illumination, and outside sunlight can be absolutely blinding. One does well to plan ahead if this is a common problem, to be well equipped with hats, sunglasses, etc., when planning outdoor activities, so that if symptoms arise, or if you notice considerable squinting, you can immediately reduce the light input to your eyes.

If this is a problem, I have one suggestion that may be helpful. Often sunglasses will reduce the amount of light reaching the eyes from directly ahead, doing little about light coming in from the sides. Of course, wraparound sunglasses answer this problem, but often cannot be worn over corrective eyeglasses.

One inexpensive solution to this irritating problem is to buy tinted safety glasses, which can be worn by themselves or directly over many corrective glasses. To find these, look in the Yellow Pages of your phone directory under "Safety Equipment." In all larger cities you can find stores that specialize in the sale of such equipment to industry, but most will sell also to an individual. Simply tell the clerk that you want to purchase a pair of tinted safety glasses. Since they are made of plastic, they do scratch rather easily, but are inexpensive enough for you to buy several pairs. Their shape, and broad temple pieces, will significantly reduce the light reaching your eyes and minimize many headache-inducing sun-bright days.

CHAPTER 10

Drugs

My view is that *drugs should be avoided as much as possible* in the control of headaches. If one is conscientious about using both systematic preventive methods and the emergency techniques shown in this system, there should be no need for drugs. However, realizing that although our intentions are the best, none of us is perfect in our execution, there may be times when an aspirin is the better part of wisdom if taken along with the other corrective aspects of this system.

However, for informational purposes, you should understand the headache drugs you may have been taking in the past, so I will discuss both proprietary and prescription drugs, in that order.

Proprietary Drugs

These are the items which can be purchased at any drugstore or supermarket, without prescription, for the relief of pain, mostly headache. Their sales add up to approximately $450 million per year in this country, *every year!* Is it any wonder that the companies making these products can afford a lot of television advertising time? The principal item, of course, is aspirin, since only 12 percent of the dollars are spent for products that do not contain this substance, either alone, or with buffers, etc. The balance of the market (still sizeable at $50–55 million) is fought over by the several sellers of acetaminophen. So let's examine these two drugs, and then the brand names concerned.

Aspirin: Americans average about one hundred aspirin tablets per person per year, for the incredible total of about twenty-two billion tablets per year! And that does not count the five hundred other medications in which aspirin is a key ingredient, such as the widely advertised buffered products.

Aspirin is an ancient drug, dating back at least to the Greeks, since Hippocrates recommended willow bark as an analgesic (pain-reliever) in childbirth. The chemical known as aspirin occurs naturally in a number of trees and shrubs, and is known chemically as acetylsalicylic acid. It was first synthesized in the 1850s by a French chemist, but, as often happens in science, was ignored until Felix Hoffman, a chemist for Friedrich Bayer & Co. in Germany rediscovered it forty years later. The Bayer Co. started selling aspirin in 1899, and it was soon put to all sorts of use as the "wonder drug" of its time. It is said to be responsible for Rasputin's power over the last czar of Russia. The physicians attending the czar's son gave him aspirin for relief of his joint pain, without realizing the danger of aggravating the boy's hemophilia, which worsened rapidly. When Rasputin displaced the physicians and their aspirin, the boy's bleeding problems "miraculously" improved. This little bit of history illustrates the greatest danger of aspirin, its deleterious effect on blood coagulation.

The exact action of aspirin in the human body is one of the great medical science mysteries, especially considering the length of time it has been in use. It is now thought that aspirin affects prostaglandins, which are hormonelike regulators that are found in almost all body tissues. This may well be the way it reduces fevers and inflammation, by blocking the formation of certain prostaglandins. But how it raises the pain threshold is not clearly understood. However, it is important to understand that in many headaches, aspirin may bring relief solely by raising your pain threshold to the point where the headache is no longer perceived, not by altering the base cause of the headache.

The hazards of aspirin are numerous, although not all individuals are equally sensitive to them. The primary hazards revolve around the effects on blood clotting and, hence, excessive bleeding, but studies have implicated it in gastric ulcers, stomach upset, and asthma. Some individuals in middle age develop what is called aspirin intolerance, in which ingestion can be followed by gasping, wheezing, and shortness of breath. There are also recent studies showing some possibility that pregnant women show increased incidence of anemia, stillbirths, and delivery complications when aspirin dosage is taken almost daily.

The effect on blood clotting is now being put to good use as several medical centers are testing aspirin for its possible long-term effects in reducing the incidence of heart attacks and strokes. Suffice it to say that you should be aware of all the effects of aspirin, and monitor your own reactions closely enough to be aware of any adverse effects it may have on you. Be particularly concerned about any marked changes in the way you react.

One last comment on aspirin, and related drugs, is that careful studies on pain thresholds have shown that two regular aspirin tablets provide all the change in threshold that you are going to get. The absorption time is roughly fifteen to thirty minutes, and the threshold will remain elevated for two to four hours. You do *not* get any faster or stronger relief by gulping more tablets or taking them at shorter intervals. It is this kind of *abuse* that is most likely to produce ill side effects.

Acetaminophen: This drug is far more familiar by the widely advertised trade names Datril or Tylenol. It is one of a group of aniline or coal tar derivatives used for some years that include acetanilid and phenacetin. It is also a constituent in Excedrin. Tylenol has been on the market more than ten years, but when Datril was introduced in late 1974, the advertising war began in earnest. Since then other entries have appeared.

This drug is both an analgesic (relieves pain) and an antipyretic (reduces fever), but it is not anti-inflammatory as is aspirin. It produces its pain reduction with one or two tablets, and taking more is both useless and perhaps dangerous, depending on the quantity and the individual. In massive doses, this drug can produce fatal liver damage; massive dose being defined in this case by as few as thirty tablets, although death rarely occurs unless forty or more are taken. Aspirin, of course, can also cause fatalities, but it is much slower-acting and gives the warnings of coma and shock. Acetaminophen is definitely a drug that should be kept away from children. However, to those who suffer stomach distress or other side effects of aspirin, acetaminophen can be an effective substitute.

Ibuprofen: This is the active ingredient in Nuprin and Advil. The drug was introduced as Motrin (prescription only) for its anti-inflammatory effects in both rheumatoid and osteoarthritis. Because of its analgesic properties, it is now produced in smaller dosage tablets for over-the-counter sales for general pain relief. Its action in the body is not well understood but, like aspirin, it is believed to reduce inflammation by its action on prostoglandins.

The fact that a prescription is still required for higher dosage tablets means that specified dosage must not be exceeded and that side effects can be significant. Ibuprofen is reported to produce less of the mild stomach distress associated with aspirin, but peptic ulceration and gastrointestinal bleeding have been reported in a small percentage of users. The manufacturer's literature states that it should not be used by aspirin-sensitive patients, or by children under 12, and stresses that it should not be used at all in the last three months of pregnancy. Thus, even for the headache sufferer who insists on an occasional analgesic drug for emergencies, ibuprofen seems to have no real advantages over aspirin or acetaminophen.

Other Compounds: The only other materials likely to appear in headache tablets are the drugs phenacetin, also known as acetophenetidin, a relative of acetaminophen, and various salicylic acid derivatives with aspirinlike action. Several also contain caffeine, which we describe elsewhere as having beneficial vasodilating effects at certain stages in the headache, but which should be used with caution where hypoglycemia may exist.

Composition of Headache Tablets

Aspirin: Normally these are 325 mg. (usually shown as 5 gr., the English unit equivalent to the metric measure) of acetylsalicylic acid. One brand is equivalent to the next insofar as headache effect goes. However, one problem with this chemical is that it is slightly unstable in the presence of moist air, and some brands will tolerate this condition better than others. Also, the bitter taste is more obvious with some brands than others, perhaps due to the rapidity of solution during the brief interval the tablet is on the tongue when being swallowed. The various children's aspirins are typically 81 mg. (1½ gr.).

Aspirin based:

Alka-Seltzer: 324 mg. aspirin, 1904 mg. sodium bicarbonate, and 1000 mg. citric acid.

Anacin: 400 mg. aspirin, 32 mg. caffeine.

Anacin Arthritis Pain Formula: 488 mg. aspirin, aluminum and magnesium hydroxides.

Ascriptin: 325 mg. aspirin, 150 mg. Maalox (magnesium aluminum hydroxide).

Bayer 8-Hour: 650 mg. aspirin with time release coating.

Bufferin: 325 mg. aspirin, aluminum glycinate and magnesium carbonate.

Bufferin, Arthritis Strength: 486 mg. aspirin, aluminum glycinate and magnesium carbonate.

Cope: 421 mg. aspirin, magnesium and aluminum hydroxides.

Ecotrin: 325 mg. aspirin, coated to dissolve in small intestine.

Empirin Compound: 225 mg. aspirin, 155 mg. phenacetin, 32 mg. caffeine.

Fizrin: 324 mg. aspirin, 1450 mg. citric acid, 1825 mg. sodium bicarbonate, 400 mg. sodium carbonate.

Persistin: 488 mg. salicylsalicylic acid, 155 mg. aspirin.

Acetaminophen based:

Bromo-Seltzer: 325 mg. acetaminophen, sodium bicarbonate, citric acid.

Datril: 325 mg. acetaminophen.

Datril 500: 500 mg. acetaminophen.

Excedrin: 97 mg. acetaminophen, 130 mg. salicyamide, 194 mg. aspirin, 65 mg. caffeine.

Excedrin P.M.: 500 mg. acetaminophen, 38 mg. diphenhydramine.

Panadol: 500 mg. acetaminophen.

Percogesic: 325 mg. acetaminophen, 30 mg. phenyltoloxamine.

Tylenol: 325 mg. acetaminophen.
Tylenol, Extra-Strength: 500 mg. acetaminophen.

Ibuprofen based:
Advil: 200 mg. ibuprofen.
Medipren: 200 mg. ibuprofen.
Nuprin: 200 mg. ibuprofen.

Prescription Drugs

This section will be brief for two reasons. First, if you are taking prescription drugs, you must be under the care of a physician, and he should answer detailed questions about your prescriptions, especially as they relate to you. Second, I am generally opposed to the use of strong drugs in the treatment of headaches. Obviously, there will be some exceptions to this, but, in general, drugs for headache relief have almost no more effect than placebos.

There are basically three groups of drugs that may be prescribed for headaches. One is the addicting analgesics, which include natural alkaloids such as morphine and codeine; derivatives of these such as Dilaudid; and synthetics that act like morphine, such as Demerol and a host of other trade names. One drug I would include in this group is Darvon, a derivative of methadone known chemically as propoxyphene. Although Darvon is sold as a nonaddicting analgesic, much recent evidence refutes that description. It not only may be addicting to many users, but has never been shown to be any more effective in pain relief than aspirin. I would strongly recommend against the use of Darvon for headaches. The important factor in all of these is the word "addicting"; that should be warning enough for anyone!

The second group of headache drugs would be those specifically for migraines, starting with the old standby ergotamine. This is a strong vasoconstrictor, that is, it shrinks down the arteries of the head, thus reducing the pressure on the nerve endings in those arteries. That is the same effect, of course, that my system will produce *without* drugs. Other drugs aimed specially at migraines include Sansert, Deseril, Sandomigran, Periactin, Demigrana, Catapress, and perhaps the second most popular, Inderal, a trade name of propranolol, a drug first used for angina pectoris, the pain of coronary heart disease. All of these, and others, show some improvement with some patients, but there is no cure-all.

The last group is the tranquilizers, for which I have great distaste. *Probably no group of drugs has done so much harm to so many people.* I'm not speaking of the disasters of birth defects, or actual fatalities, but of the kind of living death for some, where these drugs (especially if taken with alcohol, as is often the case) reduce the person to an inoffensive vegetable. True, tranquilizers make the violent more manageable and cushion the perception of life's trials and tribulations, but at what a price for so many. The pressure to be able to simply ignore the irritations of modern living has produced parents who are so spaced-out, so alienated from their children by drugs, that it is no wonder the youngsters regard pill-popping as the natural solution to all problems.

Some of the tranquilizers also have muscle-relaxant effects, and this is often the only reason they are effective in headaches. But if this approach is needed on an emergency standby basis, there are excellent muscle relaxants that do *not* possess the psychic effects of the tranquilizers; these will break up the tension cycle without the unfortunate side effects.

Just keep firmly in mind that all of these drugs either elevate the pain threshold or modify the muscle tone of the artery walls or skeletal muscles. *Each of these objectives can be achieved by nondrug methods.*

CHAPTER 11

How to Do It

The Specific Program

Now that you have a firm understanding of the real causes of the pain of your headaches, here is the detailed program that you must follow every day to end your headaches. There are three parts to the program.

First, and most important, is the part which you must do *every day.* I cannot over emphasize the importance of that phrase *"every day."* You must instill this pattern into your everyday life so that you would no more omit the key parts of your headache-prevention program than you would omit eating or sleeping.

The *second* part of the program consists of the detailed methods that you selected from the many recommendations of the previous chapters as particularly appropriate for your own problems, circumstances, age, physical condition, etc. Obviously, the victims of hypoglycemic headaches must put restrictions on their diet that others will not need. You must determine how you personally react to the methods. I would not expect the older victim to start inverted positions, but rather emphasize activities like walking.

The *third* part of this program involves the detailed emergency methods for aborting your oncoming headache, should one appear. Once you get into the daily system for even a few weeks, you will rarely need these, as the incipient headaches will come less and less frequently. Still, we are all human, and the tendency is to "slack off" the program after it is really successful, allowing bad habits to creep back in. Then the "stopper" methods are priceless. They are invaluable not only because they can stop the headache, but especially because *you know* they can stop the headache. Therefore, they stop the *fear* of the headache.

PART I.

The Daily Program—Every Day You Must Do:

1. Brush massage
2. Face/scalp & neck/shoulder movements
3. Spinal stretch
4. Alpha rhythm or other relaxation method
5. Posture "awareness" checks

If you do these *every day,* your headaches will stop. It is that simple. You must accept that fact, believe in it, and act on it. Please review the chapters on these specific methods, but let me review them briefly here.

1. *The brush massage: to be done every morning and every night.* It is the cornerstone of your program. If you have not yet obtained a brush, use the fingertip massage, which must be followed by the fingernail massage, as it is vital that you achieve both the deep and surface stimulation. However, I urge you to obtain a brush as soon as possible; the benefits of the brush massage are of the greatest importance to the elimination of your headaches. Remember to start the massage at the corner of your eye, and work the area in front of and behind the ear most carefully. Review the diagram showing the brush massage pattern (page 55) and memorize it. Use it, enjoy it, and you will look forward to it regularly!

2. *The face/scalp and neck/shoulder movements: to be done every day.* The object here is to achieve continual flexibility and looseness in the muscle tissues most closely related to your headaches. Although these movements seem numerous at first glance, they can be done very quickly once the sequence is understood and learned. Since they are best done in

front of a mirror, they form a natural addition to your morning grooming.

3. *A spinal stretch or straightener: to be done every morning.* It is your choice as to the exact method, depending upon your personal preferences and circumstances. I personally prefer stretching in a traction collar, and have done so every morning for years. The next best method is certainly the floor body alignment, as described in the chapter on spine straightening. This can be quite brief (although keep in mind that longer is better), and should be done before dressing to allow full freedom of body alignment without constraint from any tight clothes. When this is repeated daily, the muscles steadily regain their proper alignment.

4. *An alpha rhythm session should be part of your daily program.* The timing of this is open to your personal choice. Many will find that their "alpha" is a perfect break in the middle of a hectic day, rather than starting out first thing in the morning with it. Others may find it the perfect way to end a day, relaxing with it before going to sleep at night. A few of you may find the alpha process hard to "get with." Do not force it. Reread the chapter on relaxation, and select another method to be a part of your daily program that will give you the much-needed isolation from the cares of the day. The object is to interrupt the intensity that we headache victims invariably carry with us, to create an emotional as well as a physical relaxation. With patience and practice, you can learn to "turn off the world."

5. *Posture "awareness" checks are required every day.* Copy or photocopy the "Reminders" pages in the back of this book. Post them where you will encounter them regularly, making sure that you take a moment several times a day to review your exact posture at that exact minute and adjust accordingly. Remember: *think tall—think loose!*

PART II.

Your Personal Selections for Your Program:

You can do these either daily or several times a week, depending upon your selections. If you choose a modified diet related to your headaches, you should, of course, follow it every day. I strongly advocate general exercise, which can be done several times a week, but is far more beneficial if at least some effective exercise is done every day. (Once-a-week exercise is almost useless.) If you include one of the inverted positions, it is also something that should be done every day.

Most headache victims tend to be very time-structured individuals, so you will find that there may be complications if you detail too long and involved a daily program. You will find it difficult to maintain the program, and, what is worse, you will feel very guilty about missing all or part of it. This is self-defeating, and part of the syndrome we plan to break up.

Please understand that you need to do no more than the brief daily program specified in part 1 to decrease your headaches. This will require less than ten minutes a day, and you *should* feel guilty if you miss that. The other parts of your program, with one exception, are for your pleasure and relaxation and should be enjoyed as such. However, their inclusion will most certainly accelerate your rate of improvement. The one exception is diet. If you are hypoglycemic or have a food allergy, you must adhere to your nutritional plan with religious conviction.

Another aid that you may choose to use is the cervical collar. Many of you with tension headaches, or tension-related migraines, will find the cervical collar a great benefit. Initially you should use it for a short time every day, to help release tensions in the neck and shoulder structures. As you become more familiar with your body alignment feedback from using the collar, you can then begin to use it on a "need" basis. That is, when you sense fatigue creeping into the neck muscles or (as your sense of good posture improves) when you feel your head slipping forward or tilting back on your neck, then wrap on the collar. Even a few minutes of its support will often bring amazing relief. It breaks up the vicious circle of tension and strain, reorienting the whole head-neck-shoulders relationship, so vital to your headache-prevention system.

One last method to be recommended for your daily schedule is one of the acupressure points. The "shinbone" point, located in detail in the acupressure chapter, is not only effective against headaches specifically, but is the point that is considered to serve as a general "tonic" for your entire system. Stimulation of this point tends to normalize the entire nervous system and bring it into harmonious adjustment.

PART III.

Methods of Warding Off Oncoming Headaches:

These are vital to your success during the early weeks, before my system has had time to restructure your headache syndrome. Again, there are certain methods that you should invariably use when a headache threatens and some additional methods that you may choose personally to add to your repertoire.

The premium methods are the acupressure points and the trapezius massage. First, because they are extremely effective in stopping headaches, often almost immediately; and second, because they can be done under almost any circumstance of work and/or social life. Other emergency methods should be used as you see fit, and according to your personal preference. The brush or fingernail massage is a great "stopper," as is an alpha rhythm session, if opportunity permits its use.

Remember, any one of the many methods described can be done in a very short time. If you choose to use one that is best not done in public, such as the scalp calisthenics, it can be quickly done during a brief visit to the restroom.

Please review the secondary tools already described, and you will see how many preventive actions you can take when a headache threatens. *Know them and use them. They are functional—they work!*

Emergency Aid Reminder

At the first sign of a headache, choose from the methods described in Part III (the prime "stoppers") according to your circumstances at the moment. Your personal choice will depend on whether you are at home, at work, traveling, socializing, vacationing, entertaining, etc. Of first importance is to immediately start using your "bag of tricks," knowing absolutely that they will stop your headache!

Acupressure: can be used quickly and easily almost anywhere, anytime (even while driving). Extremely effective, so use it *immediately* when you suspect a headache.

Trapezius Massage: once learned, can be a "lifesaver," especially with tension headaches (and it feels so good!); use it often.

Fingertip and Fingernail Massage of Head: second choice to brush massage, but use whenever you can't brush. Remember to stimulate with both fingertips and nails, as described in Alternative to Brushing section.

Face and Scalp Calisthenics: great while driving, but otherwise you may want a little privacy; very beneficial.

Neck and Shoulder Rejuvenators: superb for work break. Remember to do slowly, with fluid motions; benefits body alignment as well as headache.

Orthopedic Collar: a short period wearing your collar will give great relief, if your circumstances allow it.

Brush Massage: in addition to your daily session, a brush massage can nip a threatening headache in the bud; use it promptly whenever your brush is within reach.

When you have carefully studied all of these methods and practiced them so that you know exactly what to do, you will be thoroughly prepared, should the need arise, to stop your headache. For additional security, carry your emergency card in your wallet in case your memory needs a little help.

The Magic Keys

Do you remember the four magic keys to your headache prevention?

> *CIRCULATION*
> *TENSION*
> *TONE*
> *POSTURE*

Each of these has been discussed in detail in the preceding chapters, and now you understand why they are so important in your headache syndrome. The program is specially designed to markedly improve each of these elements in your body. From the first week you begin practicing the system, you will see immediate improvement in tension, muscle tone, and posture. Please be assured that the improvement in circulation, although harder to see, will certainly accompany the others, and you will soon be very aware of the improvement.

Let me repeat something written earlier about the Magic Keys: this is a "self-help" manual. I have prescribed certain specific methods that you must use every day. Please examine the other material and select methods of interest and relevance to you. Be open and willing to experiment. You know yourself better than anyone else does, so have confidence in your judgment.

With your enthusiastic cooperation, this system will eliminate your headaches!

Caution

Certain headache symptoms *may* be indications of serious conditions that should be reviewed with a physician. The National Institutes of Health lists the following as headaches that are alarm signals for prompt and thorough medical checkup:

Sudden, severe headache, "out of the blue."

Headache associated with fever.

Headache associated with convulsions.

Headache accompanied by confusion or lessening of consciousness.

Headache following a blow on the head.

Headache associated with local pain in the eye, ear, or elsewhere.

Headache beginning in an older person previously free of headache.

Recurring headache in children.

Headache at any age that interferes with normal living.

Daily or frequent headache.

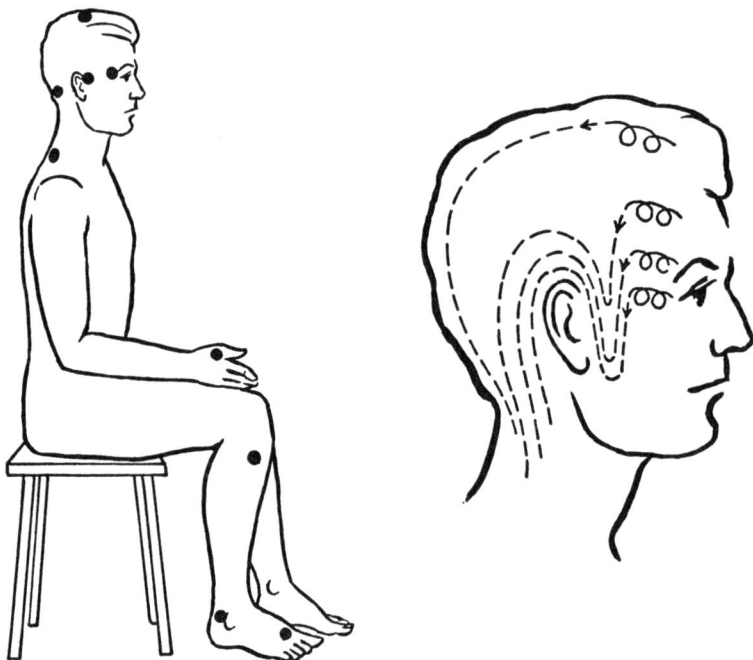

The Magic Keys

Circulation—Tension—Tone—Posture

The Daily Program—Every Day You Must Do:

1. Brush massage
2. Face/scalp & neck/shoulder movements
3. Spinal stretch
4. Alpha rhythm or other relaxation
5. Posture "awareness" checks

Face/Shoulder Rejuvenators (3x Each)
1. Eyebrows up & return
2. Right eyebrow up & return
3. Left eyebrow up & return
4. Squint both eyes closed & release
5. Squint right eye & release
6. Squint left eye & release

7. Frown deeply & release
8. Wiggle ears or scalp above ears
9. Yawn wide & close
10. Open jaw, move right & left
11. Wrinkle nose
12. Make faces!

Neck/Shoulder Rejuvenators (3x Each)
1. Both shoulders raise & return
2. Both shoulders circle forward
3. Both shoulders circle backward
4. Right shoulder up & return
5. Left shoulder up & return
6. Right shoulder circle forward
7. Left shoulder circle forward
8. Right shoulder circle backward
9. Left shoulder circle backward
10. Rotate head right & return
11. Rotate head left & return
12. Tilt head right & return
13. Tilt head left & return
14. Chin toward chest & return
15. Chin toward ceiling & return
16. Head circle right
17. Head circle left
18. Neck stretch forward & back
19. Shoulder stretch
20. Upright back stroke
21. Bend forward swimming stroke
22. Deep breathe

Sitting Posture Check
1. Weight on "sitting bones"
2. Feet on floor
3. Lower back against chair
4. Pelvis tucked in
5. Tummy in
6. Rib cage lifted

7.   Shoulders low & relaxed
8.   Check head alignment
9.   Take a deep breath—exhale
10. Tense & relax major muscles
11. THINK TALL—THINK LOOSE!

Standing Posture Check
1.   Knees relaxed
2.   Pelvis tucked in
3.   Tummy in
4.   Rib cage lifted
5.   Shoulders low & relaxed
6.   Check head alignment
7.   Shift weight foot to foot
8.   Tense & relax major muscles
9.   Flex & straighten joints
10. THINK TALL—THINK LOOSE!

These are your reminders, a key part of your self-help system for totally ending your headaches. The methods that you have read in the preceding chapters *really work*. Use them! These reminders will help in the beginning, until the methods become second nature.

Make a xerographic copy of the reminders and post them where you will definitely see them every day. The mirror in your bathroom is probably the best place.

The acupressure and emergency reminder should be carried in your wallet or purse, so that it is always available for easy and immediate reference.

Methods of Warding Off Headaches
Acupressure (esp. hands & head)
Trapezius massage
Brush or fingernail massage
Face/scalp calisthenics
Neck/shoulder rejuvenators
Spinal stretch and/or collar
Your own choices
KNOW THEM & USE THEM—
THEY WORK!

Headache Prevention Log

It is very important to keep track of your daily prevention methods. Enter the date at the left, then draw a diagonal line for each item completed. Draw a second diagonal, to form an "X," for those you do twice a day. The required daily program is printed below. Add your personal choices to the blank columns. Under "Remarks" list headaches or impending symptoms that you stop with the emergency procedures. Conscientious scorekeeping forms good habits.

Date	Brush massage	Face/scalp cal.	Neck/shoulder rel.	Spinal stretch	Alpha or relax.	Posture check			Remarks

Bibliography

Headaches

H. G. Wolff's Headaches and Other Head Pain. 3rd ed. Oxford University Press, 1972. The absolute classic of medical books on headaches, probably available only at a medical library; somewhat heavy reading.
Headaches: Their Nature and Treatment by Stewart Wolf, M.D., and Harold G. Wolff, M.D. Little, Brown & Co., 1953. The layman's version of Wolff's classic medical text on headaches. A little old, but available in many city libraries, and not really out of date.

Nutrition

You Are Extraordinary by Roger J. Williams. Random House, 1967. A beautiful presentation of why you are a unique individual.
Low Blood Sugar and You by Carleton Fredericks, Ph.D., and Herman Goodman, M.D. M. Evans & Company, 1975. An excellent book on the whole hypoglycemia syndrome and its dietary treatment and control, by a world-recognized and outspoken authority on nutrition (Dr. Fredericks), and an open-minded physician who is willing to go against the grain of the

old-fashioned medical view of this problem. Almost anyone could benefit by reading this book, since it details the problems caused by the heavy loading of sugar in the typical American diet.

Sugar Blues by William Dufty. Chilton Book Co., 1975. An excellent and entertaining discourse on the problems caused by sugar in Western civilization. Bibliography lists many related books.

Recipes for a Small Planet by Ellen Buchman Ewald. Ballantine Books, 1973. Excellent for high-protein meatless cooking.

Exercise

The Magic of Walking by Aaron Sussman and Ruth Goode. Simon & Schuster, 1967. An absolutely fabulous book about walking, and a delightful weekend's reading. If the benefits of walking described so well in the first half of the book do not turn you on to this simple but delightful form of both exercise and entertainment, the second half, a sampler of walking literature from many esteemed authors, most certainly will.

21-Day Shape-up Program by Marjorie Craig. Random House, 1968.

How to Keep Slender and Fit After Thirty by Bonnie Prudden. Bernard Geis Assoc., 1961.

Sexercises by Edward O'Reilly. Bell Publishing Co., 1967.

Adult Physical Fitness prepared by the President's Council on Physical Fitness. Sold by the Superintendent of Documents, Washington, D.C.

Adult Fitness by Fred W. Kasch and John L. Boyer. National Press Books, 1968.

Physical and Physiological Conditioning for Men by Benjamin Ricci. Wm. C. Brown Co., 1972.

Jogging by William C. Bowerman and W. E. Harris, M.D. Grosset & Dunlap, 1967. One of the earliest and finest books on jogging.

Body Alignment and Movement

Look Better, Feel Better by Bess M. Mensendieck, M.D. Harper & Brothers, 1954. The absolute classic in this field.

Body Dynamics by Gertrude Enelow. Information Incorporated, 1960.

Awareness through Movement by Moshe Feldenkreis. Harper & Row, 1972.

Miscellaneous

Renew Your Life through Yoga by Indra Devi. Prentice-Hall, 1963.

Yoga over Forty by Nancy Phelan and Michael Volin. Harper & Row, 1965.

Miss Craig's Face-saving Exercises by Marjorie Craig. Random House, 1970. Certainly lives up to its title.

Hypnosis in the Relief of Pain by Ernest R. Hilgard, Ph.D., and Josephine R. Hilgard, M.D. William Kaufmann, 1975. One of the best books available for a general review of the facts and theories of pain by two of the very active researchers in this field.

Index

A Word From The Publisher . . .

Celestial Arts is the publisher of many excellent books on health and wellness, with an emphasis on topics of awareness such as meditation, stress reduction, and spirituality. Among our finest publications are *The Realms of Healing,* by Stanley Krippner and Alberto Villoldo, as well as *Natural Vision Improvement,* the bestselling Australian book by Janet Goodrich that applies a holistic health approach to improving your vision. We also publish Michael Gach's self-help-with-acupressure books, *The Bum Back Book* and *Greater Energy at Your Fingertips.*

And we have books by Sondra Ray, Virginia Satir, Jerry Jampolsky, Barry Stevens, Richard Moss, Bob Mandel, and Emmett Miller. Of special interest is L. John Mason's *Guide to Stress Reduction,* an outstanding book on techniques of stress reduction, complete with exercises.

For a complete list of our books, please write for our free catalog or call us: CELESTIAL ARTS, P.O. Box 7327, Berkeley, CA 94707, (415) 524-1801.

A Word From Ten Speed Press . . .

Celestial Arts is a part of the total publicatuin program of the publishing house *Ten Speed Press,* publishers of such fine books as *The Wellness Workbook, High Level Wellness,* and *What Color Is Your Parachute?* Please write or call for their free catalog: TEN SPEED PRESS, P.O. Box 7123, Berkeley, CA 94707, (415) 845-8414.